Same Storm Different Boats

Covid, Community and How We Come Together

Jason Strelitz

Oakamoor
Publishing

First published in 2025 by Oakamoor Publishing

Woodside, Oakamoor, ST10 3AE, UK

ISBN: 978-1-910773-95-6

A CIP catalogue record for this book is available from the British Library.

Oakamoor Publishing's Editorial Review by Dr Charlotte Woodcock

Cover image by Grant Gilbert

ACKNOWLEDGEMENTS

The thanks for this book go deep and wide. In a leadership role, you stand on the shoulders of the hard work of so many people, and their creativity, passion, skill, persistence and graft. Just the people I worked directly with during the Covid period numbered in the hundreds, including amazing colleagues across Newham Council and the NHS, many in the voluntary sector, community and faith organisations, community champions, and other lay community members. I name a few people across the book, but for the many more unnamed, I hope you know how much I recognise you, too. I hope you see this book as a fitting account.

The whole public health team in Newham were extraordinary, facing this unprecedented career challenge together, speaking to each other morning, noon and night, pushing themselves to their limits, and all with a spirit of collaboration, kindness and humour.

There are also many people who supported me deeply during this intense period. In particular, I would like to acknowledge Kevin Fenton, a font of wisdom and generosity; my direct manager Colin Ansell, who gave me all the freedom and autonomy I wanted to bring creativity and ambition to my work, and all the support I needed to know he had my back (plus share a good few jokes along the way); Althea Loderick, chief executive of Newham Council at the time of the pandemic, who brought a calm leadership from which I learned so much; Mayor Rokhsana Fiaz, whose limitless drive and ambition for the borough, and deep passion for equity and social change, helped drive my own beliefs in what we could and should strive for; my fellow Directors of Public Health, grappling with similar challenges as myself, from whom I learned so much, and many of whom always provided a willing ear for advice and support. I would also like to thank Jo Cleary for her support for me personally, and our public health team, particularly when things were hardest.

The idea to turn this experience into a book was fuelled by a few presentations I gave as the pandemic wound down. In particular, talks to the Jewish Medical Society and at the Centre for the Analysis of Social Exclusion at the London School of Economics, where I had done my PhD 20 years before, gave me the sense of a story I wanted to share. As the book began to be drafted, I was grateful to be hosted at the Centre for Social Policy for a seminar, and a detailed reading by Roger Bullock.

Several people commented on drafts. I am deeply grateful to them for their time, kindness and thoughtfulness. Lucy Easthope, Carolyn Wilkins, Julie Billet and Barry Quirk, all people from whom I have learned a lot about leadership; Ruth Hutt, a peer who played a similar role in Lambeth during the pandemic, and who I admire immensely; and Gidon Freeman, a dear friend who gave me a valued lay perspective on a story I hope is of interest to people with broad social interest.

I am deeply grateful to Leslie Turnberg who read my draft with deep interest and recommended me to James Lumsden-Cook, his publisher. In turn I'm very grateful to James for his belief and commitment to this book and his colleagues at Bennion Kearny who patiently edited my drafts.

Finally, I'd like to say thank you to my amazing family and friends; to my soulmate Mandy Wilkins, my unflinching rock of support, professional and personal, my principal reflector on life's many challenges and sharer of life's joys; and to Matti and Tami, now so grown up from their pandemic days, who did not get all the attention they might have got from me at that time, but were wonderful and inspiring throughout and ever more so today.

CONTENTS

Same Storm
Different Boats

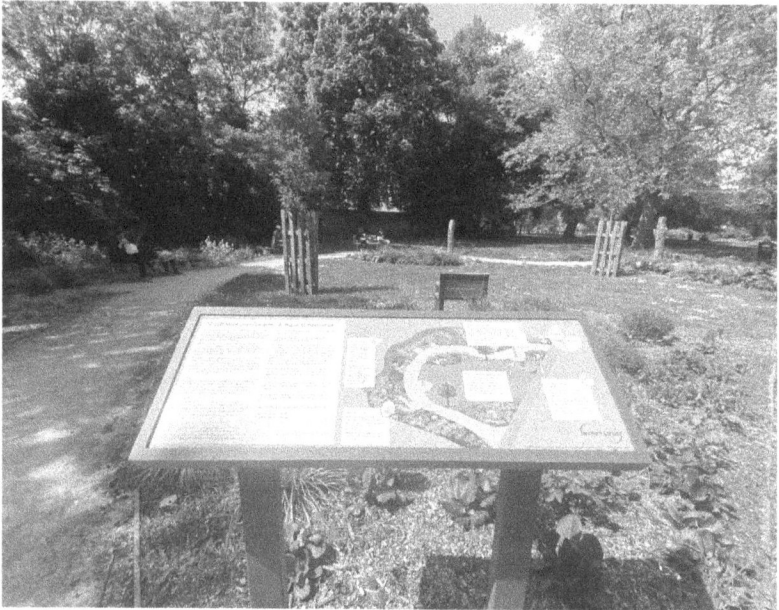

*Newham's Covid-19 Memorial Garden in Plaistow Park
in memory of those who lost their lives during the pandemic
and to honour the frontline services and volunteers who
supported the borough's most vulnerable residents throughout.*

Chapter 1

"Everyone Has a Plan Until They're Punched in the Mouth"

Mike Tyson isn't an obvious person to start a public health story with, but I've yet to find a quote which better summarises how I felt about my Covid-19 experience.[1] The Covid pandemic was the time in our lives when plans went out the door. Plans for holidays, plans for family celebrations, work plans, school plans. Across the UK and much of the world, it was a time of plans being cancelled, and their replacements cancelled once more.

But the former heavyweight champion's words also speak to me professionally – to our pandemic plans. Our plans for a major flu outbreak had been gathering metaphorical dust somewhere on our public health hard drives, waiting for this moment, and yet no sooner had Covid got underway than we found them totally inadequate for what was unfolding. That wasn't because it was a coronavirus rather than the flu; it was because next to no one could imagine a virus totally taking over our lives, society, and economies in the way that it did, in a matter of weeks. Throughout the next 18 months, more plans would have to be made to cover approaches to testing, the shielding of clinically vulnerable people, contact tracing, and outbreak management. Often, they would be changed again, within days, by adjustments in policy, genetic variation in the virus, or some other factor.

I should remember when I first heard about Covid-19, just as I remember other significant, tragic, global and national moments: when 9/11 happened, 7/7, the Grenfell Tower

---

[1] Throughout the book, I generally use the shorthand "Covid" for brevity unless there are particular reasons to refer to Covid-19 or Coronavirus.

Fire disaster. But I don't. The journey into Covid happened in slow motion at first. Initially, it appeared as an emergent virus in Wuhan Province in China, not a place I had heard of before. On January 4th 2020, the World Health Organisation (WHO) shared news on Twitter of a cluster of cases of pneumonia from Wuhan, with no reported deaths. A week later, the WHO issued a statement saying, *"No clear evidence of human-to-human transmission of the novel coronavirus."*

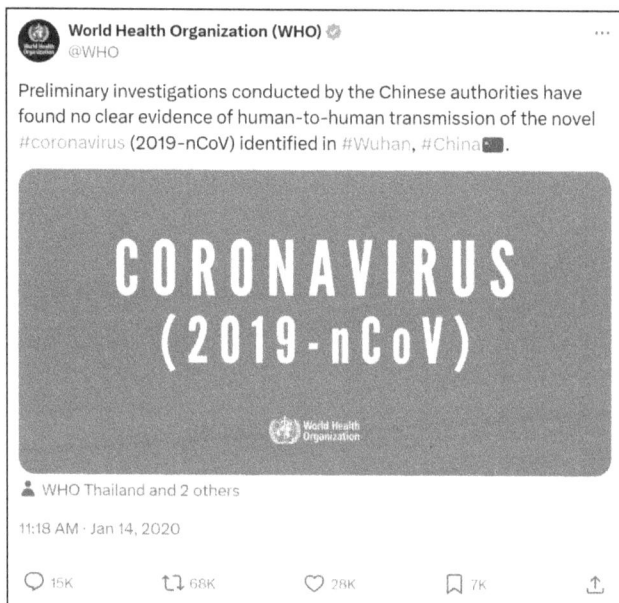

World Health Organization (WHO) ✔
@WHO   ...

Preliminary investigations conducted by the Chinese authorities have found no clear evidence of human-to-human transmission of the novel #coronavirus (2019-nCoV) identified in #Wuhan, #China▪.

CORONAVIRUS
(2019-nCoV)

World Health Organization

👤 WHO Thailand and 2 others

11:18 AM · Jan 14, 2020

💬 15K   🔁 68K   ♡ 28K   🔖 7K   ⬆

But things were starting to escalate quickly.

As the month went on, what was happening in China seemed straight out of Hollywood movies like *Outbreak* (incidentally, most of my friends thought this was what my job was like) when it actually bears almost no resemblance to Hollywood fiction. What was real, what was not? How much did the particularities of China – with censorship and the difficulties of reporting – cloud our understanding of what was really going on? Whole towns were being constrained in their daily movements due to the virus. Really? OK, but this is China; they operate by different rules.

It was another month before the first case was identified in Italy. That started to change perceptions, but only partially. The scenes on the news were awful: people crowded on trolleys in hospital corridors and despairing dispatches from Intensive Care Units, scenes of police guarding the outskirts of villages so people couldn't leave, significant levels of death and distress. All this in a country that I know, a place I've been to several times, and much more similar to our own life in the UK. Yet, somehow, what was happening still seemed distant, too fantastical to be true, too unimaginable to believe that it might be coming here and turning our lives upside down.

Until it did.

Even as late as March 13th 2020, just ten days before the UK's unprecedented lockdown, the BBC published an optimistic article online: *Coronavirus: Three reasons why the UK might not look like Italy.*[2]

Although I can't remember when I first heard about Covid, I have my notes from my initial meeting about the emergent virus in late January 2020. I have the first briefing I did for the mayor and local politicians, where I was working as director of public health in Newham, East London. I can see in my diary when I had my earliest briefing with the Chief Medical Officer (CMO) Chris Whitty, soon to be a household name thanks to his regular appearances by the side of the Prime Minister, explaining the latest epidemiology (the pattern of the outbreak). In time, he would even have his own catchphrase – "Next slide, please" – and become, no doubt, the first CMO to make the social leap from providing

---

[2] Coronavirus: Three reasons why the UK might not look like Italy, BBC News, https://www.bbc.co.uk/news/uk-51858987

scientific advice to government to spawning coffee mugs with his face on them.

I remember when I called my team together to say we were dropping everything we were doing and that Covid was our only priority for now. Then, I have the thousands of emails and WhatsApp messages that followed as the avalanche of Covid reality hit us month after month after month.

For so long, we had no idea how the pandemic would ultimately play out; wave after wave of strains of Covid caused infections and loss, but as widespread vaccination finally offered protection to our society, both in the UK and globally, the world was able to move on.

Writing in 2025, five years on from the start of the pandemic, Covid – as a significant part of life – has now slipped into the past. When it comes up in conversation, I and most people I talk to, see that period as some kind of surreal dream/nightmare. It was so very real, and sustained, but it also feels like an oddly detached moment; as if it was a glitch in the "space-time continuum", as Doc Brown from *Back to the Future* may have said. Occasionally, I might hear a friend or colleague who sneezes (and has tested) say, "Oh, it's not Covid," but mostly it doesn't get mentioned anymore.

Unless a new strain emerges that significantly withstands the protective effect of vaccination, with hospitals overflowing once again, we have moved into a period of acceptance. Covid is a new health risk, alongside the others that we simply live with. For those interested, whether from a policy perspective or those who lost loved ones and still want some answers and understanding, the UK Covid-19 Inquiry presses slowly forward. Chaired by Baroness Heather Hallet, this gargantuan piece of work will provide a thorough analysis of the UK's pandemic preparation and immediate response, and hopefully provide us – as a country – with valuable lessons for the future. Others battle personally with the effects of Long Covid. The long-term impact on our National Health Service remains profound, too.

For me, personally, the pandemic period will undoubtedly remain one of the most extraordinary periods of my professional life, and those of my team and many peers. As a director of public health, I went from a bit-part player – part analyst, part agitator – a fairly peripheral leader in local life, to being at the centre of it, trying desperately to help my colleagues and my community navigate a storm. Alongside local political leaders and other colleagues, I helped lead one area's response from day one, all the way through to the end. I chaired multiple meetings a day, briefed politicians, addressed virtual community meetings, and appeared on TV and radio to try to communicate what was going on in our area and the challenges we faced. I led and supported an astonishing team of public servants for whose work ethic, values, skill, creativity, and humour I will forever be grateful. I worked harder than ever before, slept (even) less, worried more, cried, got angry, but also found joy and laughter, too.

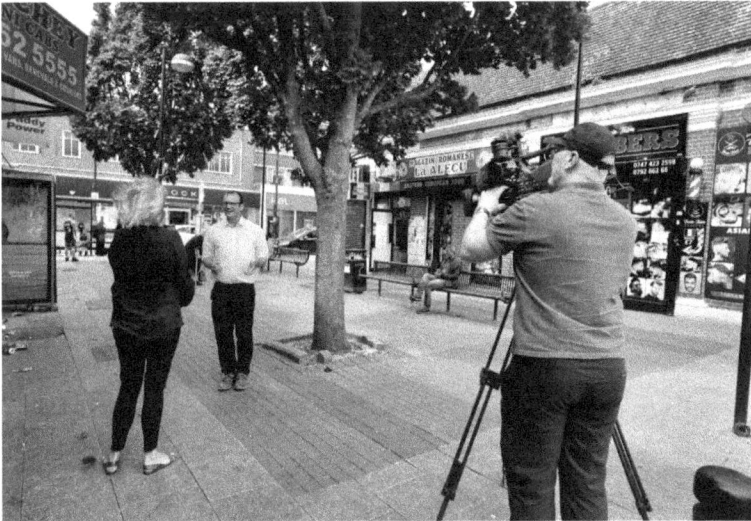

One of many TV interviews; here promoting the NHS App, just off Green Street, Newham.

As well as being a pandemic professional, like everyone else, I was a pandemic participant, parent, and partner. Uniquely, this event touched us all, and my work life was intertwined with the experience that we all had, through the lockdowns, the creation of bubbles, the long-awaited plans cancelled, and the loneliness and dreariness of the second lockdown of winter 2020-2021.

But I was very fortunate, as well. Those closest to me were spared by this awful virus; I didn't endure close family and friend loss and the inability to grieve properly that so many did. I was also privileged in my lifestyle, a home where people could work and have personal space, with computer devices for all to support our new online life, and takeaway treats to break the monotony. In my personal life, everyone stayed mentally well, despite the obvious reasons for despair. My work in East London, a place where so many of these things could not be taken for granted, reminded me to appreciate those privileges daily.

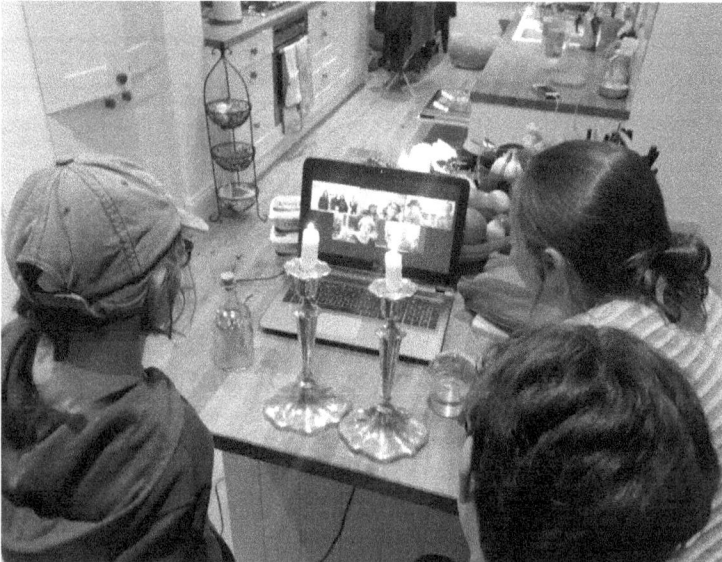

An everyday pandemic moment; marking the Jewish Sabbath on Friday night with my family on Zoom.

But the privilege I want to share in this book was my being at the centre of this event. As a professional participant, albeit at a very local level, I was involved with every aspect of how one area – and in my view a particularly fascinating place – was impacted and responded to this extraordinary period.

I want to explain why a place like Newham (and many places with similar characteristics) was so affected, the way Covid had a magnifying effect on inequality, and our understanding of it. I want to shed light on the community's resilience, how people came together to try to weather this storm, where the strengths emerged from, and to share what it felt like as national debates raged but then played out at a local level. In doing so, I think there are important insights to emerge from the pandemic period. Not just those that the inquiry will focus on in terms of pandemic preparedness and response, but much more broadly about community and inequality in the UK today. As the world faces ever greater economic and social instability, from climate change to economic disparity and conflict, how do these impact our least-privileged communities, and how can we work together to build our collective resilience not just for future pandemic events, but through the everyday challenges that our unequal and increasingly unstable world throws up?

The scale of loss from Covid can be hard to digest, and each death was a profound loss to those impacted. However, in their totality, the numbers tell a profoundly important story. Our Newham pandemic timeline, overleaf, plotting key moments in the pandemic against the daily death and confirmed case total, gives a sense of the journey that I, and those I worked with, travelled. Two dramatic and devastating peaks sit within the first half of the timeline, pockmarked with a flurry of activity and intervention. A further confirmed case peak emerged at the end of 2021, the beginning of 2022.

The first wave mortality peak coincided with very few confirmed cases, as testing was barely available other than for those admitted to hospital.

The second mortality peak was matched by a huge increase in confirmed cases as there was widespread access to testing in the community, with both PCR (the original laboratory-based testing) and increasingly lateral flow testing (the home tests).

The third visible peak was the Omicron/Delta variants case peak. This time, however, with a widely vaccinated population, the link between cases and mortality had been broken. Living with Covid became increasingly realistic. Over later months, a small but consistent mortality picture endured, though increasingly not matched by a significant confirmed case rate. We knew that large numbers of people did continue to have Covid, but increasingly – in the absence of a nationwide testing infrastructure – we relied on other sources such as the self-report ZOE App and the Office for National Statistics surveillance study to understand the quantity.

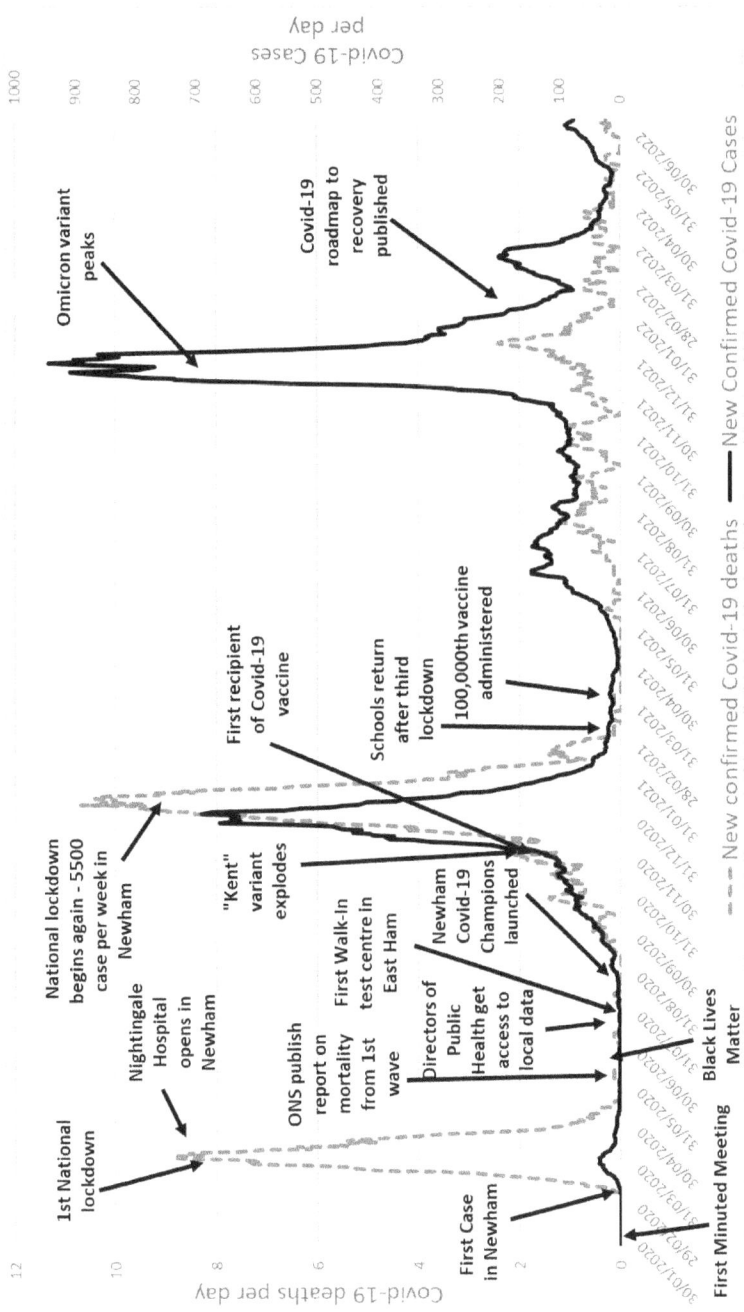

New Covid-19 cases and deaths (7-day average) in Newham throughout the pandemic.

It was in late September 2021 that our public health team gathered in person for the first time in 18 months. Like many people, we had worked intensely through the period, but in back-to-back Zoom conversations, rarely seeing each other in the flesh. We rolled out two long sheets of lining paper and marked out the months of the pandemic in marker pen. We handed out Post-it notes and – for an hour – we wrote down all the things we had done to try to support our community to navigate the challenges of Covid as safely as possible.

We had set up a network of community testing facilities, a distribution service that redirected surplus food to those who needed it, vaccine clinics in mosques and gurdwaras, community "digital inclusion hubs" for people who lacked digital access to get online, and volunteer befriending services so that people weren't isolated.

We had also provided advice and guidance to places of worship, businesses, and schools so they could operate as safely as possible, outreach teams to reach those living on the streets, and Champions networks to galvanise the power of community.

In turn, we had piloted the NHS Covid App, developed a contact tracing and welfare service that would call everyone who tested positive in the borough to link them in with medical and social support, developed hotel isolation facilities so that those in overcrowded and multigenerational homes were not forced to spread the virus at home, and supported Eid prayers for a large Muslim community to take place in our parks so that people could celebrate safely.

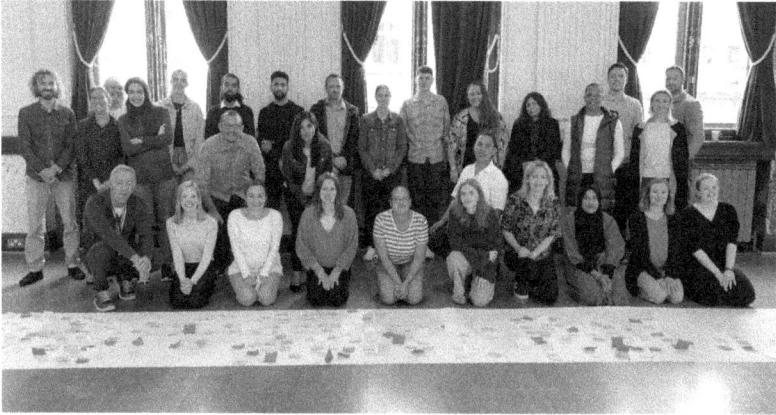

Newham's Public Health team gathers towards the end of the pandemic to reflect on our journey, with our timeline of activity.

There was so much to be inspired by – amazing collaboration with the community, extraordinary innovation catalysed by pressing need, and almost all at a breakneck speed, atypical of local government's reputation or, fairly typically, reality. We gained important insights into the obstacles and constraints faced by the less privileged inhabitants of Britain, as Covid exposed the realities of poverty and unequal employment experiences, housing, education and health, of racism and the experience of many people from black and minority ethnic communities.

I do not cover every aspect of the response to the pandemic in this book. Many people were intensely involved in responding to Covid, but in very different ways to me: doctors and NHS professionals, scientists, care workers, and lots of my local government colleagues. Even my peers doing the same job as me – in any of the 150 local authorities around the country – will have experienced many similarities but also differences in where the pandemic took them, and where the needs of their communities meant different experiences, impacts, and responses.

The book follows the pandemic broadly chronologically. I begin with an introduction to my discipline – public health – and my role as a local government director of public health, plus an overview of the fascinating place where I work, Newham in East London. Each subsequent chapter focuses on a theme, exploring the nature of the challenge and the response through my personal experience. In doing so, I will touch on the work that many colleagues led. The book reflects my perspective on these events and my views, and in no way is supposed to represent the views of colleagues, Newham as a place, or directors of public health more widely.

This is my account.

Chapter 2
A Director of Public Health 101

A widely used definition of public health is *"The science and art of preventing disease, prolonging life, and promoting health through the organised efforts of society."*[3] Explaining what that means – in terms of my job as a director of public health – in a comprehensible way to people outside my field is not totally straightforward. Before the Covid pandemic, it is fair to say most people had no idea. In trying to make sense of it, I came up with the following explanation.

A doctor's role is to see an individual, diagnose what is wrong with them, and if necessary, together with the right experts, treat them with medicines and other technologies. In contrast, the job of a local government public health professional (in much of history, and still in many countries, the senior ones are medically trained) is to understand the main health issues facing a particular place and work to address them. That could be anything from imminent health threats (like a pandemic) or more commonly longstanding issues like chronic diseases. Understanding patterns, *who* is affected, to *what* degree, and *why*, is our profession's underpinning science, known as epidemiology.

With that understanding communicated to the relevant people, our role – together with everyone who can make a difference – is to develop and implement strategies to improve the health of the local population based on those priorities. Since its foundation, which I will come to, public health has always placed a strong emphasis on approaches to prevent ill health in the first place. So, prior to Covid, as a director of public health, I led a team which worked on

---

[3] What is Public Health? - FPH - Faculty of Public Health

prevention strategies targeted at a wide range of health issues my community faced, including diabetes, young people's mental health, and the health of homeless people. I worked with medical professionals, but also schools, housing professionals, businesses, charities, leisure providers – whoever had the potential to make a difference. Critically, public health work also means working with politicians, whether nationally or locally. Public health is political in nature; if doctors are making individual clinical decisions about the treatment of patients, public health decisions are about policy choices and investment decisions. These, ultimately, rest in the domain of political leaders.

One of the animating insights of current public health practice, both in the UK and globally, is rooted in the work of Professor Sir Michael Marmot, with whom I worked earlier in my career. His research has focussed on the "social determinants of health" and has shown, using an overwhelming evidence base, that the health differences in people from different backgrounds are largely rooted *not* primarily in their access to, and experience of health services, but social factors: *"The conditions in which we are born, grow, live and age,"* as he writes.

Marmot asks us to consider not just the "causes" of ill health but "the causes of the causes" to really understand the fundamental drivers. One of the original pieces of research that shed light on this insight was the Whitehall Study that began in 1967, following thousands of civil servants across different pay grades. At a time when many thought that health differences between people from different backgrounds were likely driven by the risks associated with manual and white collar work, the Whitehall Study showed clear distinctions in cardiovascular health for civil servants at different grades, with those on the lowest grades faring worst.[4] That was despite all these individuals working in office-based jobs. The conclusion? There must be factors at play other than the blue collar/white collar distinction.

Marmot has repeatedly shown what is referred to as the *social gradient* in life expectancy. Women growing up in the 10% most deprived areas of England can expect to live for nearly eight years fewer than those in the most affluent 10%; for men, the difference is nearly ten years. With modern medicine, our 21st-century healthcare is very good at keeping people alive but much less good at ensuring they are healthy. So, the gap in healthy or disability-free life expectancy (how many years of good health someone is expected to experience) is even steeper, with an average gap of 12 years between the least and most deprived areas, and up to 20 years at the extremes.

The next figure shows healthy life expectancy for every local authority area in England and where that area ranks in terms of the government's measure of area deprivation. As is evident, the correlation is strong and clear-cut: in England's poorer areas, people spend many more years of their lives in poor health.

---

[4] M. Marmot, et al. (1991) Health inequalities among British civil servants, The Whitehall II Study, *The Lancet*, June 1991.

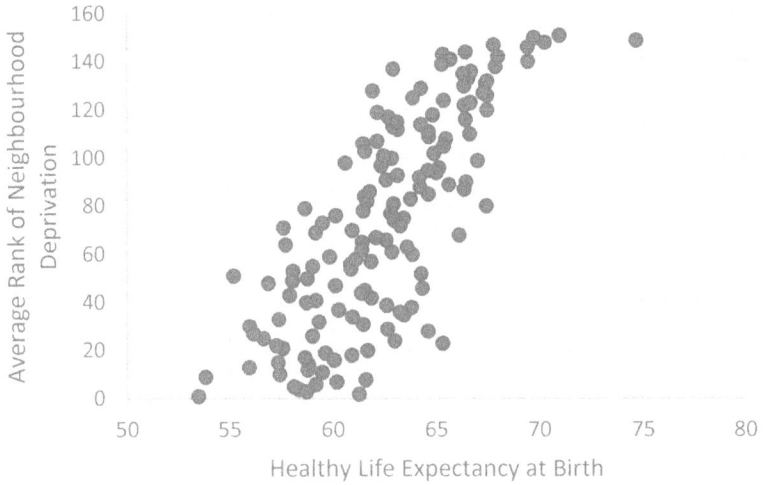

Healthy Life Expectancy at Birth and Area Deprivation.
Source: ONS (2018-20) / Index of Multiple Deprivation

Given this evidence base, public health focuses relatively little on 'medical treatments', which research shows account for a minority of the difference in health outcomes across a given society, including the UK. Although there are important inequalities in access to healthcare in the UK, the National Health Service – for all of its challenges – ensures that at a basic level, from maternity care through to child health, mental health, emergency care, and the treatment of long-term conditions and the illnesses of ageing, access to treatment is not dependent on income or background. Private healthcare, by comparison, accounts for a very small proportion of UK healthcare, although this proportion has been rising in recent years.

Linked to this and public health's focus on prevention is a deep concern with *health inequalities*, a fairly esoteric term that refers to the unequal health outcomes observed between different parts of the population in a given place. Most typically, these are discussed in terms of differences in life expectancy; for example, between certain cities and towns, neighbourhoods, or different ethnic groups. Thanks to careful and detailed research, we understand these differences as social in cause and, therefore, preventable and amenable to social solutions.[5]

The existence of health inequalities or the pursuit of health equity (as many prefer to term it) is a moral cause. Why, in a rich society, should someone's social circumstances determine such large differences in something as fundamental as how long they live? For many who work in public health, this injustice is what motivated us to work in the field. Many are moved by the line Marmot used in publishing his report for the WHO on global health inequalities: *"Social injustice is killing people on a grand scale."*

But beyond the moral case, given the cost to society of these inequalities (such as years of lost productivity and costs to the state like social security) and given that they are preventable, there is a strong case for policymakers and the voting public to be concerned about them.

'Health inequalities' has remained, as I mentioned, an esoteric concept, rarely registering much with public consciousness (moments in the pandemic being an exception), and occupying an uneasy relationship with policymakers. The first major policy report on health inequalities, led by Sir Douglas Black (a doctor and President of the Royal College of Physicians), was commissioned in 1977. Published in 1980, not long after Margaret Thatcher's new government had come to power, the receiving Secretary of State, Patrick Jenkin, wrote the foreword to the report. Highly unusually for such a report, he threw it under the bus.

"The group (that had written the report) has formed the view that the causes of health inequalities are so deep-rooted that only a major and

---

[5] WHO Commission on the social determinants of health.

wide-ranging programme of public expenditure is capable of altering the pattern (of health inequalities)... I must make it clear that additional expenditure on the scale which could result from the report's recommendations – the amount involved could be upwards of £2 billion a year – is quite unrealistic in present or any foreseeable economic circumstances."[6]

And then, the most stinging rebuke.

"...quite apart from any judgement that may be formed of the effectiveness of such expenditure in dealing with the problems identified. I cannot, therefore, endorse the Group's recommendations."

The report was quietly published by the government on a Bank Holiday Monday, and only 280 copies were printed.

Thirty years later, a similar pattern would follow. The government commissioned a new report on health inequalities towards the end of the 2000s, led by Marmot himself, entitled *Fair Society, Healthy Lives*. It was written in the shadow of the financial crisis of the late 2000s and published in February 2010, three months before a general election.

This time, it would land not with explicit rejection, but into an environment of sustained public spending austerity and a commitment to reduce the size and scope of the state. With significant parallels, Marmot commented on how little the government has followed the evidence set out in his report in the ensuing years.

Of course, inequalities would gain greater significance as the pandemic wore on, and are central to this book.

---

[6] Inequalities in Health: Report of a Research Working Group (1980).

Changing Emphasis

Demographers refer to 'epidemiological transition' when (in a given society) the burden of disease switches from infectious diseases to chronic diseases of ageing and lifestyle as that society becomes more affluent. This is where we are in the UK. As such, the focus of much of my work is the killers and disablers of today: cancers, cardiovascular disease, mental ill health, and their causes. This contrasts with many developing countries, such as Malawi where I have spent time, where infections and "communicable diseases" – those that pass from one person to another – still represent a significant burden of disease.

However, even in societies that have gone through this transition, infections and communicable diseases remain important in our public health professional DNA and our roles as protectors of the population's health. This is partly deeply historic; our profession's founding moment is the widely known story of physician John Snow, who removed the handle of a water pump in the slums of Victorian Soho to end a cholera epidemic.

What led to that moment was what we would now call "community engagement" and "disease mapping". Snow went from home to home to ask people about their symptoms, *when* they had become unwell, and *what* they had done before becoming ill. He turned those conversations into data, mapping the epidemiology of the infection, and used the information to challenge the accepted orthodoxy that cholera was spread by miasma or bad air (the origin of the word malaria). His approach – to gather evidence, use it to challenge current thinking, and apply it to action – would become the hallmark of the public health methodology.

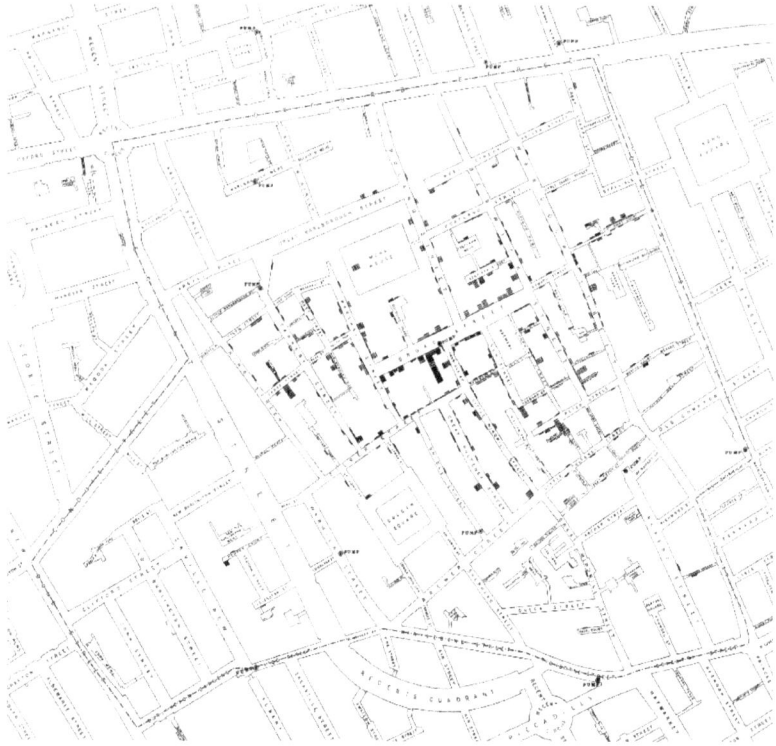

John Snow's map of Cholera cases in Soho, 1854.

Shortly afterwards came one of the great public health advances: the development of the sewerage system. It is a historical oddity that this immense leap forward – an obvious response to Snow's scientific advance – occurred only by chance. The sewers were commissioned because of the big stink in London and, therefore, as a solution to the smell and miasma causing disease; Snow wasn't yet believed. Unwittingly, however, the sewers worked, and cholera, typhoid, and typhus were reduced significantly in the city, and public health action was happening at scale.

I'm regularly reminded of this history when I cycle to work. After passing London's 2012 Olympic stadium, I ride past Abbey Mills pumping station in Newham, one of Joseph Bazalgette's extraordinary buildings that powered the original sewerage system and remains in operation today. Known historically as the "Cathedral of Sewerage" for obvious reasons, I'm told that local kids prefer the name "Poo Palace".

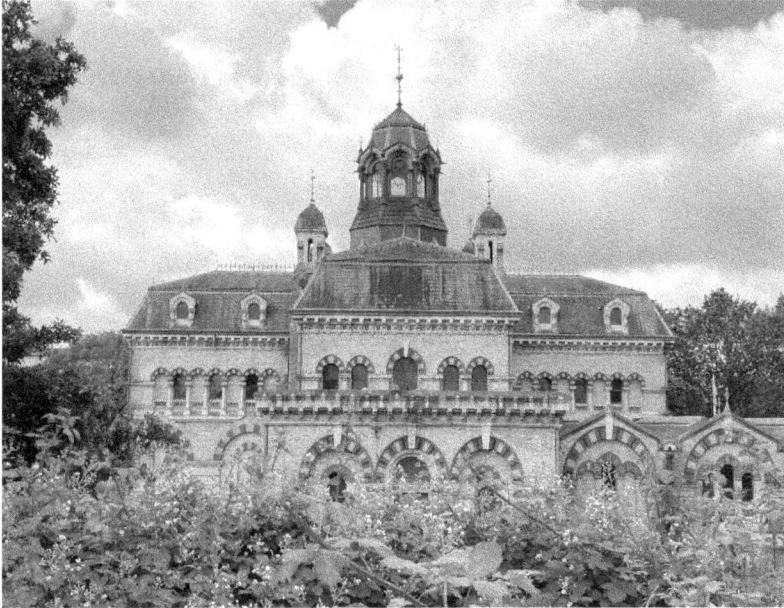

Joseph Bazalgatte's Abbey Mills Pumping Station – "Poo Palace" – as viewed from my cycling commute, Stratford, Newham.

Another leap forward in public health, which is also relevant to the Covid story, comes from the same period. The 1840s saw a greater understanding of the link between a poor environment and health. Edwin Chadwick, a social reformer who, like Snow, used research to inform and underpin his work, campaigned for the 1848 Public Health Act, which would eventually lead to strong local government involvement in public health for a century. It would also lead to the creation of inspectors of nuisances, who would eventually become today's environmental health officers

(EHOs), much-valued colleagues before, during, and since the pandemic.

The importance of infectious disease control to the public health profession also has more recent resonance. The HIV epidemic was the major public health crisis of the late 20th century and is well within the professional memory of public health practitioners. Since the start of the epidemic, HIV has caused over 20,000 deaths in the UK and 40 million globally. The fact that this killer passed among seemingly healthy people posed an enormous challenge for scientific understanding, community engagement, stigma battling, and the support behind behaviour change. HIV/AIDS has had a profound inequalities dimension, too. Through the worst years of the epidemic in the UK – the 1980s and 1990s – it impacted the gay community heavily, and over time had an enormously disproportionate impact on the global South. The immediate health risk – HIV/AIDS – was a virus (i.e., a biological exposure), but the nature of its impact, affecting different communities hugely unequally, had a greatly social dimension; the "causes" and "the causes of the causes".

Training

The importance of infections and communicable diseases in the history and present day remit of public health means that the management of infectious diseases and other environmental hazards is a key part of public health practice and training: a specialist area typically referred to as health protection.

In training, I spent considerable time on this, largely managing isolated incidents and small outbreaks of measles, norovirus, legionella, food poisoning, or other incidents that arise in wealthy countries (mostly relatively low-impact infections, in part due to widely available vaccination, clean water, food safety and antibiotics). I learnt the basics of contact tracing, trying to understand how particular infections spread between different people and how public health works to identify the causes of outbreaks before implementing measures to break an infection's ongoing transmission and spread.

The very beginning of my public health training in 2009 coincided with the H1N1 "swine flu" epidemic. Although the impact in terms of mortality was substantially less than initially feared, it was a major public health challenge that required huge mobilisation. I was a total novice to public health, a junior at the start of my public health journey. I was responsible for carrying out very basic tasks, contributing to the wider effort, but had little understanding of the broader context of what was happening and how my work fitted in.

Fast forward ten years, and I was just nine months into my first job as a director of public health. Infectious disease control, not my natural strength, had barely touched my radar for years. We still tried to ensure high levels of vaccination, particularly for childhood diseases, and the rollout of the newer HPV vaccine for teenagers, and unlike most parts of the UK we also still worked on tuberculosis (TB). This disease, largely absent in much of the country, remains present in Newham and some other inner urban areas, characterised by high levels of migration from TB-prevalent regions around the world. Largely, however, our focus was on the chronic physical and mental health issues facing more affluent societies.

A couple of months before Covid arrived, I was at a workshop for a small number of new directors of public health from around the UK. Tracy Daszkiewicz, who had been director of public health in Wiltshire when the Novichok poisonings had occurred, was sharing her experiences with us (she was portrayed later by Anne-Marie Duff in the BBC drama *The Salisbury Poisonings*). I reflected in the discussion with her that – in all likelihood – someone in the room would face a *major* public health crisis of some sort in their career. After all, in the previous few years alone, Tracy had to tackle the challenges of Novichok, and other colleagues around the country had faced the aftermaths of the Manchester bombings, the Grenfell Tower fire disaster (where I had worked, too), and the London Bridge attack. As it turned out, within a couple of months, all of us in that room would be knee-deep in the largest, most acute public health crisis in the UK for a generation. The role of director of public health was coming to the fore…

Chapter 3
Newham, East London

The idea of 'place' is central to public health.

Every community – through its population, character, resources, assets, and social and health challenges – reflects its particular demography, socio-economic circumstances, culture, and history. In order to give meaning to the story of Covid in Newham, it is therefore vital to share some of its history and distinctive characteristics. Its current character has roots that are hundreds of years old, but is also marked by multiple transformations, not least since it hosted the Olympic Games in 2012.

Newham is an East London borough formed by the merger of East Ham and West Ham in the 1960s. It is, along with its neighbour to the west, Tower Hamlets, the heart of London's old East End.

Bounded by the River Thames to the south, Newham's growth was tied to the docks, like the Royal Albert and Royal Victoria docks, and factories further north. The Tate and Lyle sugar refinery and factory opened on Plaistow Wharf in Silvertown in the 1880s and still produces over a million tins of Lyle's Golden Syrup each month, a legacy of that shipping and industrial heritage.

From the 1960s onwards, London's docks, unable to manage the new container-laden cargo ships, began to close. Slowly, over the next two decades – as across London as a whole – factory production also ceased and London transitioned, painfully at first, from an industrial to a service economy. Newham was also notable for its stars of England's 1966 World Cup win. West Ham's Bobby Moore, Geoff Hurst, and Martin Peters are immortalised (along with Everton's

Ray Wilson) with a statue on Barking Road, near West Ham United's old ground off Green Street.

Already a home for many immigrants to the UK (there were once, for example, five synagogues in the borough, reflecting late 19th and early 20th-century migration from Eastern Europe), Newham has increasingly become a favoured landing point for many new arrivals with cheaper housing compared to much of London, and burgeoning communities of fellow migrants. Large populations came from India, Pakistan, and Bangladesh, and there is a long-standing community of Caribbean origin.

Over time, many of the old East End pubs slowly disappeared and, in their place, sprang up an array of places of worship – mosques, gurudwaras, temples, and evangelical churches – plus eateries and grocers catering to people from around the world. Newham became one of the most multicultural areas in the country, full of vibrant neighbourhood centres, such as East Ham High Street, Green Street with Queen's Market, Canning Town, Stratford, and Forest Gate, to name just a few.

The Newham of today is truly multicultural, with no dominant groups and over 100 languages spoken. Many new arrivals come from South Asia, alongside significant communities from West and East Africa, China, Eastern Europe, and many other parts of the world. John Marriott brilliantly captures the multiculturalism in his encyclopaedic history of the East End, *Beyond the Tower*.[7] Speaking of where he lives in Manor Park, in the North East of the borough:

"Opposite is a superstore, owned and run by Gujarati Hindus which sells the cheapest rice and spices in the area, while a little further down Romford Road is the Turkish Istanbul, grocer for fresh fruit and vegetables at any time day or night. My hair is cut by Iraqi Kurds, my

---

[7] J. Marriott, *Beyond the Tower: A History of East London*, Yale UP, 2012.

car fixed by Sikhs, take away meals are provided by a Pakistani shop, most of my domestic repairs are done by Polish builders and internet facilities are offered by Somalis. Within 150 metres of my house are a Nigerian episcopal church, a Bangladeshi Mosque, a Tamil mandir, a Sikh gurudwara and a Baptist community centre."

A version of this could apply to almost anywhere in Newham.

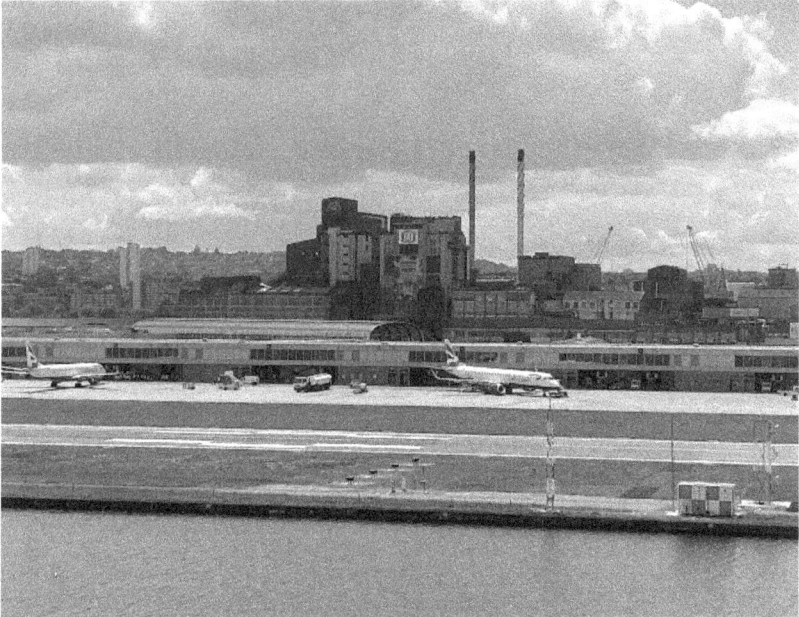

Newham old & new: Tate & Lyle Sugar Refinery since 1880 with City Airport in the foreground.

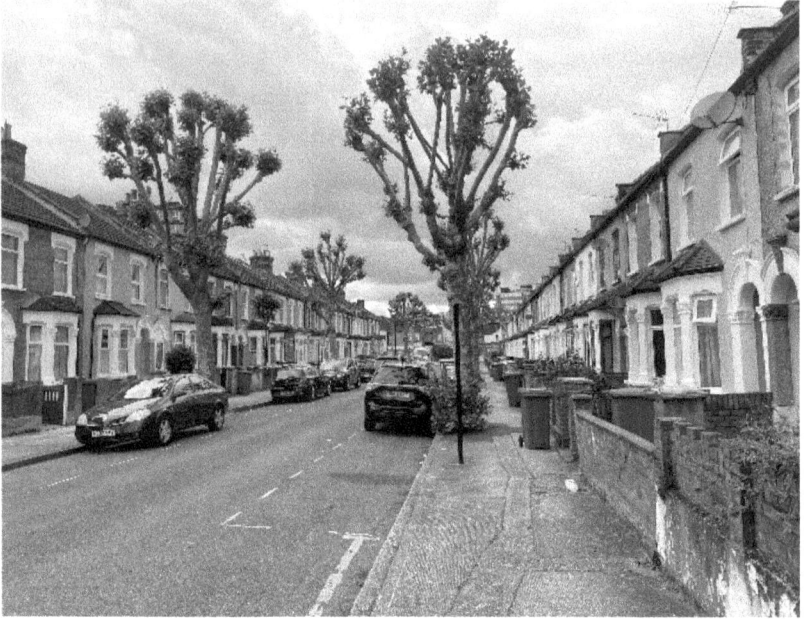

Typical Newham Terrace, Plaistow.

At the last census, in 2021, 45% of households had at least one person for whom English was not their main language, the highest percentage anywhere in England, and 1 in 5 households had no one for whom English was their main language.

While there has been a continuing secularisation of majority British cultural life, organised religion and prayer remain a significant part of life for many ethnic minorities. In Newham, 85% of people say they have a religion, among the highest proportion in England and Wales, and compared, for example, to 45% in Brighton, 58% in Nottingham, and 76% in Birmingham.

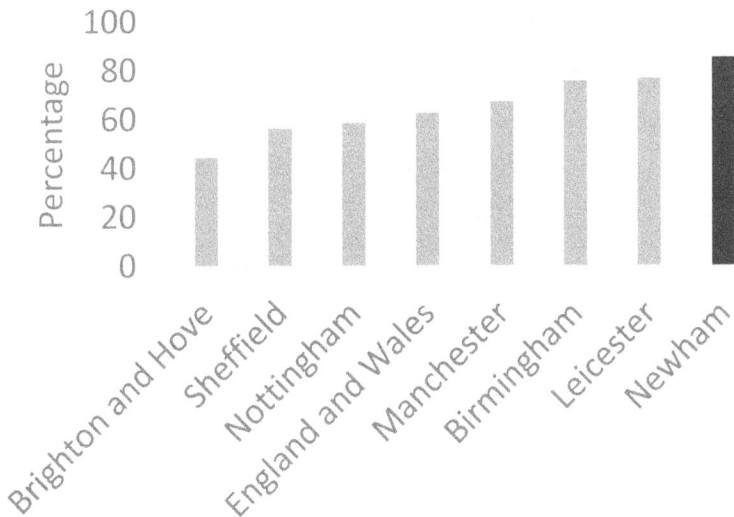

Percentage of population who state they have a religion, selected cities and England and Wales. Source: Census 2021.

Despite working in these kinds of areas for many years and being from a religious background myself (though not personally religious), it was something I had never really engaged with professionally, until I worked as part of the Grenfell Tower fire disaster recovery. There, in my role as public health consultant, trying to understand the ways in which the disaster had affected the local population to help inform a plan for recovery (the epidemiological impact), I saw the centrality of mosques and churches in people's lives in the response to the disaster and the community's recovery. This is definitely the case in Newham.

It's not just identity, though. The many places of worship throughout the borough are hugely important parts of the social fabric of the area and people's daily lives.

Newham was the host of London's 2012 Olympics, and the Olympic Park was developed mostly on the land of old factories and disused sites in Stratford, alongside the huge new Westfield shopping complex that sprang up over the same period. These brought new assets to the area and jobs for local people while driving an increase in house prices much later than in many other parts of London. This brought about a further population shift with large numbers of long-standing homeowners cashing in on their new property gains and moving out of the area, as well as a significant increase in private landlords.

These changes in population continue. There are stable, long-standing communities in Newham, but also huge population mobility, with a significant turnover of residents on an ongoing basis. There are large numbers of students, including many thousands coming from overseas, at local universities such as the University of East London, based in the borough, and more recently, a campus of University College London. As a community of communities, Newham is a place where many refugees and asylum seekers come, as well as others with uncertain immigration status. At one stage of the pandemic, a local piece of research estimated there were 10,000 people in the borough described as "having no recourse to public funds", a status given to migrants in the UK who do not have permission to settle for a given period of time, which leaves people destitute.

Newham has an extremely young population, far younger than most parts of the country but more typical of areas with large ethnic minority communities. It has excellent schools and an aspirational population, with many young people entering higher education (large numbers use local universities or great institutions across the capital).

Alongside the vibrancy, aspiration, and community vitality, there is plenty of poverty. Despite Newham's proximity to the glass buildings of Canary Wharf and the City of London, the wages of the local population are well below the London average. Much of the population is in service occupations, such as transport, care, retail, and security.

Newham has proportionately more people renting homes from private landlords (as opposed to owning their homes or living in social housing) than almost anywhere else in England. On its own, this is neither good nor bad. On the one hand, it provides people who need it with flexible housing options, but on the other hand (and for many), it means poor conditions and a level of community instability. With low-income families prioritising cheap housing, landlords don't always have an incentive to invest in decent property conditions. Moreover, there are very high levels of overcrowding; by some distance, the highest levels of any local authority in the country. Whereas around 1 in 50 households are crowded for the country as a whole, in Newham it is more than 1 in 5. The housing situation has also left the community vulnerable to the more recent cost of living crisis, which we shall return to later, as rents have risen far quicker than wages.

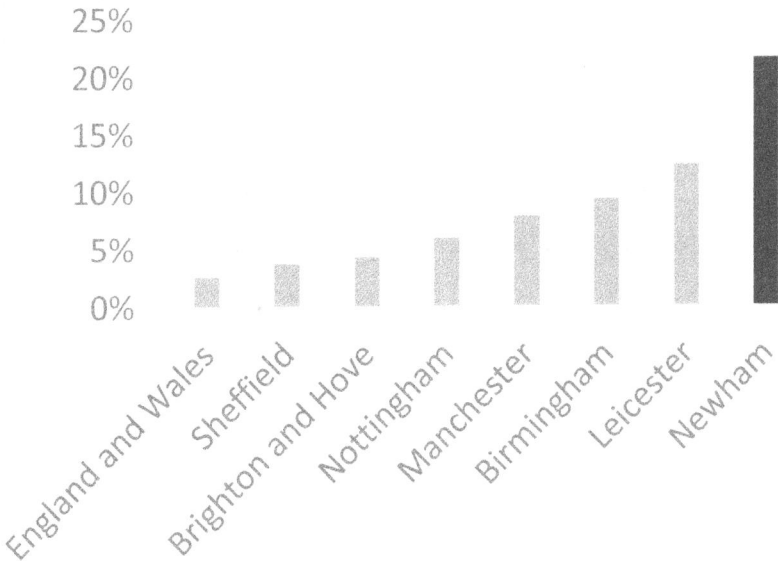

Percentage of population who live in overcrowded housing, selected cities and England and Wales. Source: Census 2021.

This pattern of housing makes the borough feel different from other urban areas I know and have worked in. The poverty in Newham is less obvious as it does not have the large areas of tower blocks and sprawling housing estates found in many other London boroughs. Newham's poverty is more hidden in the overcrowded Victorian terraces that line many of the streets, away from the shiny new towers of the recently gentrified areas in the west of the borough.

These conditions of poverty and poor housing, as the evidence from Marmot and others would suggest, contribute to deep underlying health inequalities. On average, people in Newham live shorter lives than those in many other places in the UK and enjoy good health for fewer years. The inequalities in health can be seen from maternity and early childhood through to old age and across many different aspects of physical and mental health (the links between poverty and poor health are many and varied).

There are particularly high levels of cardiovascular risk in Newham's population. The combinations of poverty and the ethnic makeup of the population create a risky cocktail of factors. Undoubtedly, the way we eat in our calorie-rich, time-poor societies means that healthier food is more expensive, which drives people on lower incomes to the fried chicken shops that saturate Newham's high streets and offer filling £2 meals.

Poverty limits not just available resources but also eats into both time (people working long and inflexible hours) and personal resilience (which many of us need to draw on to retain a semblance of a healthy diet). Poverty also impacts the other side of the energy equation – calories burned. With less money and time to fit in exercise, and similar resilience required, being active is also harder. Few people these days are doing physically demanding jobs. And the environment matters, too. Newham's streets are congested, its pavements narrow, and its air quality very poor. The ability to be active

in daily life – by walking, running, and cycling – is also limited.

The links between poverty and cardiovascular risk are also compounded by ethnicity. The precise factors that explain these relationships are not clear, but it is likely that there is a combination of biological factors, such as a genetic component of how metabolism functions, the conversion of energy from food in our bodies, and social factors linked to stress. Whatever the combination of reasons, the risks are strong. Diabetes, for example, is far more prevalent amongst people of South Asian heritage than the White British population and hits people at a much younger age.

As I wrote at the start of this chapter, in public health, place matters. This combination of factors – closeness of community, the nature of work, the type of housing, patterns of family life, and underlying poor health – would provide a potent environment for Covid to cause particular tragedy.

Chapter 4
The Arrival

January 31st 2020

It feels painfully naïve now. After my first minuted meeting about the 2019-nCoV Wuhan novel coronavirus at our local Newham Borough Resilience forum, I wrote the first of what would be hundreds of briefings to Newham's mayor, other local politicians, and senior leaders.

"Two patients in England have tested positive for Coronavirus; they are both well and specialist measures are in place to prevent the spread of the infection."

Looking back, it was not that the threat was not being taken seriously; it was just that the arrival of Covid coincided with what felt like much bigger news. Indeed, my above note went out on the same day that Brexit happened – the end of the painful, all-consuming chapter in our history when the UK officially left the European Union.

Looking back at the news clips from the time, it's easy to see where the tone of my briefing came from. The mood was one of concern, but of things also being under control; the specialists in serious infectious disease control knew what to do. We recognised that the first two cases presented us with a challenge, but at that time, few saw them as canaries in the coal mine warning of impending doom.

The gears seemed to be barely shifting at this stage.

A couple of days later, I attended the first of what would become regular confidential briefings for directors of public health with Chief Medical Officer Chris Whitty. These briefings would become invaluable over time, a safe space in which the CMO – in his calm, wise tone – would honestly share his assessments of the current situation and, as directors of public health, we could ask him questions. Over time, I would learn a huge amount from the CMO himself, as well as my exceptional peers in the same role around the country. Nevertheless, this was just the beginning, the very earliest days of trying to understand what was going on. For me, from a non-medical background and no expert in respiratory viruses, my instinct was to try to understand the emerging picture while taking a lead from more experienced and expert colleagues.

Over the next few weeks, things seemed to develop very slowly. While my diary was pockmarked with the odd Covid briefing and updates, it was mostly business as usual – the normal range of planning meetings, community visits, and budget discussions. I was taken on a tour of the incredible developments at the Olympic Park, with a new university campus, alongside museums and galleries sprouting up in this once anonymous corner of London. I visited a community organisation revitalising East London's historic waterways from their post-industrial past. Each visit was punctuated with tentative, speculative conversations about what this virus would mean for us in the UK.

One notable action from this period was reviewing our pandemic influenza plan. Looking back now, this was – for many reasons – of limited use in the situation we found ourselves in (not simply because it was for influenza rather than a coronavirus). There are important arguments to be had elsewhere about preparedness and good plans at a national level, but this requires a separate discussion and will no doubt be the subject of much debate following the publication of the Covid-19 inquiry.

The next meaningful act was our first support for one of Newham's many communities, in this case the small local Chinese community. In the earliest days of the pandemic, with the focus on Wuhan, we were dealing with both anti-Chinese racism that was creating understandable concern, and a need for infection control advice within the Chinese community. Our positive local relationships in Newham meant that, as Chinese New Year approached, we were in a good position to support the leader of the Chinese community association, Gill Tan, one of the hundreds of community "low-flying" heroes we built relationships with over the next 18 months.

This period also coincided with the February half-term school holiday. There were active debates in the public health community about what should happen when Covid was clearly impacting Northern Italy, and the ski holiday season meant that many people would be travelling to that region. No controls were put in place.

Imagine trying to grow a lawn, putting your hands into a bag of seed, grabbing handfuls and scattering them over the grass. Infectious disease specialists borrow the term "seeding" to describe the landing of a virus in a place and the process of it spreading. That is what was about to happen on a significant scale. People newly returned from abroad, particularly those heading to Northern Italy for a skiing holiday, would "seed" the virus across the UK. That spread would initially be particularly concentrated in London for obvious economic and social reasons.

I continued to be mostly reassured by the messages coming from senior policymakers. However, I was starting to hear other perspectives, too. One of my oldest friends, a GP in a much more affluent part of London, was worried and thought policymakers were not seeing what was going on. With a much larger group of patients who had been, or would know people who had been, to Europe in half-term, he was concerned that he was seeing and hearing about lots of potential cases. Without testing in place, those fears could not be confirmed initially; the clinical early warning system was going unnoticed.

That's the key thing about these first weeks of the pandemic in the UK. As a country, we could have acted more quickly based on clear evidence from other countries. However, policy felt like it was being driven only by what we could see in *our* data. Dissident voices emerged, but the partial data picture had a powerful impact on perception, and our own data was open to criticism.

1. We were doing barely any testing. Initially, the only testing was happening in hospitals, so the only real cases we knew about were those who had become seriously unwell and been admitted. A study by Imperial College in 2021 estimated that, in London, 2% of cases in the first wave were being admitted to hospital. This is called the Infection Hospitalisation Ratio, and this was lower in London than the national average because of London's younger population.[8] If that was the case, in all likelihood, possibly 50 times the number we knew about were actually infected; they just weren't ill enough to be in hospital. The test criteria soon expanded to include a small amount of community testing, focusing on people who had both symptoms and a particular travel history. It would be a long time (in epidemic terms) before there was any significant level of testing.

2. There was a time lag between when someone became infected and, if their condition deteriorated, their hospital admission. Epidemiologists started to understand the pattern of infection and disease progression in both China and Italy. After someone became infected, there would be an incubation period, the period before symptoms start to develop. Symptoms would then emerge and, if they were

8 Edward S. Knock, et al., Key epidemiological drivers and impact of interventions in the 2020 SARS-CoV-2 epidemic in England. *Science Translational Medicine*, 13.602 (2021).

unlucky, these would persist and the person's health would deteriorate, and they would be admitted to hospital. Only then would they be tested, and by the time the test result came back, it might well be a couple of weeks since they had become infected. In the UK, we were judging the current state of a rapidly escalating epidemic based on a highly limited slice of data that was – at best – two weeks old!

3. Finally, guidance started to emerge about staying at home if you had symptoms. However, a huge amount of Covid infection was being passed from person to person, with the initially infected individual (host) displaying no symptoms at all. (Like many children, my daughter, who was ten at the time, picked up an amazing pandemic lexicon, including the phrase "asymptomatic transmission".)

Therefore, on April 3rd, in what would turn out to be the peak of the first wave in Newham, there were only 60 confirmed cases in the borough. By comparison, on January 3rd 2021, the peak day of the second wave, when community testing was widespread and readily available, Newham had over 1,000 confirmed cases, but we will come to that much later.

So – to circle back – action in this first phase was based on a tiny slice of limited and highly misleading data.

March 13th 2020 – Our First Confirmed Case in Newham

A week earlier, I had met a much more experienced colleague from another borough for coffee. How serious was this thing, we deliberated. We still weren't sure. How did it compare to the swine flu outbreak we had been through ten years previously?

The number of cases had been steadily rising for a couple of weeks. At first, directors of public health would receive a call from Public Health England, the arms-length government body responsible for infectious disease control (which was disbanded during the pandemic and replaced by, amongst other bodies, the UK Health Security Agency), to say they had a positive case in their area and that they must plan appropriate infection control measures.

Every day, I waited; surely it couldn't be too long before I got a call? Newham is normally first in the line for health challenges, often for all the socially determined reasons discussed earlier, we sit at the wrong end of health league tables, from immunisation rates to diabetes prevalence. However, with a local population far less likely to have been to Europe to enjoy alpine ski resorts over half-term, we would wait a bit longer. I couldn't quite believe that – every day – we seemed to dodge the bullet, as colleagues around London were being called into crisis meetings. In turn, I was starting to understand what was happening, but only at a tentative, basic level. I still had no comprehension of the scale of what was unfolding, but I started to tell colleagues and our local politicians to assume that Covid was in the borough and that it was a question of *when* not *if* it would be confirmed.

Despite that, that first case was significant when it came. That was partly because it just made things very real. Every step in those early stages felt like a psychological tennis match between the awful picture we could see from oversees, and this calmer – although for the reasons described above – highly misleading picture we had in front of us. But it was also significant that it took so long for the first confirmed case in Newham. By the time our first case was substantiated, Public Health England had abandoned its policy of phoning directors of public health to alert them. I found out about our first case the same way everyone else did, by clicking refresh on a publicly available government data dashboard at just after 5 pm, when it updated.

Over the next few days, we would see a case here, a case there, but we hadn't yet internalised the insights from above about why the low case numbers were misleading. There was no social distancing at this time. Two days after our first case, Google asked its employees to stay at home, marking the beginning of active measures by a small number of corporate employers, but these initial steps were marginal in the scheme of things. In essence, Covid was spreading unchecked.

This was still the situation by the second week of March 2020, six weeks following my first meeting about Covid and three weeks after the end of the half-term holidays. There were no general restrictions on mixing. Yes, people with certain symptoms were asked to stay at home (and a cough may have got you a concerned look in the aisle in Tesco), but other than a focus on hand hygiene and cleaning surfaces, and a move from handshake or hug to fist bump and then elbow touch, there was still a real sense of life carrying on as normal.

With these limited changes to behaviour, we were actually in a period of completely out-of-control spread, an invisible exponential growth in numbers… a ticking time bomb.

As I began to attend more meetings with colleagues, and started to follow emerging debates among experienced infectious diseases epidemiologists on Twitter, I developed an understanding of the toolbox we would have to control the emerging epidemic. In particular, I became newly familiar with the concept of "social distancing", the different potential permutations of distinct policy approaches, and the wider impacts these may have.

By mid-March, I was surprised that some social distancing measures had not been brought in. I recognised that these were difficult decisions. The modelling from epidemiologists like Dr Neil Ferguson at Imperial College, London, was quite terrifying, and to a degree just unimaginable; he predicted that an uncontrolled Covid epidemic could result in as many as 500,000 deaths (the death total would end up being roughly half that figure). There was now increasing evidence to suggest that the UK would not somehow miraculously avoid this storm.

The government argued for delaying the introduction of major behavioural restrictions based on a belief in the concept of "behavioural fatigue". The argument was that the impact of restrictions on people's freedoms would progressively diminish over time as people would increasingly stop complying at some point. Thus, it was better to delay any restrictions until an optimum moment. This did not make a lot of sense to me. I searched for evidence to support this fatigue logic and could not. However, even accepting that there was a plausible rationale for this position, I considered that surely a relatively small percentage of people getting tired of rules at the end of a period of restrictions (when hopefully the epidemic had significantly slowed) would be less impactful than nobody facing restrictions when the epidemic was escalating.

With the virus now circulating freely and quickly, the vulnerabilities of Newham and other similar places would be laid bare.

We typically think of community as a positive entity and protective for health – providing social connection, solidarity and support – and there is plenty of evidence to support this. Nearly 100 years ago, the Peckham Experiment was launched in South London, promoting the idea that by nurturing community in a place with high levels of poverty and disadvantage, people's health can be improved. More recently, building on the pioneering work of sociologist Robert Putnam, including his influential book *Bowling Alone*, an increasing wealth of evidence has demonstrated the health-promoting power of social capital, networks, and community. The WHO has asserted that loneliness, for example, is an equivalent health risk to smoking 15 cigarettes per day (community can also create the conditions in which adverse health behaviours are normalised).

Undoubtedly, though, the strength of the community in Newham at this early point in the pandemic, rather than being protective, actually posed an additional risk. With religious life carrying on as normal, people of all ages were filling the mosques, churches, gurdwaras and temples of Newham. These places, indoors and full of singing and communal intimacy, were perfect spreading environments. I saw it with my own eyes in my own community, the Jewish community of North London. Here, religious life was carrying on as normal, too. The festival of Purim, a celebratory day of fancy dress and dancing, fell on March 9th, and synagogues were as busy as ever with families of all ages. Add to this the weddings, funerals, and other customary rituals of communal life, which were going on as usual. The community was paying a hidden toll, which would only become apparent weeks later. In Newham, one of the most religiously observant parts of the country, Covid was undoubtedly spreading rapidly.

This spread, though, was not simply due to a lack of awareness and delayed action, although the lockdown would dramatically curtail it. Many risk factors for the transmission of Covid were linked to unavoidable aspects of daily life: the jobs people do, the homes they live in, the buses they travel on, and the high streets where they shop. These factors would make it harder for the community to protect itself throughout the rest of the epidemic, even when, over the coming months, the risks and possible mitigations became more apparent.

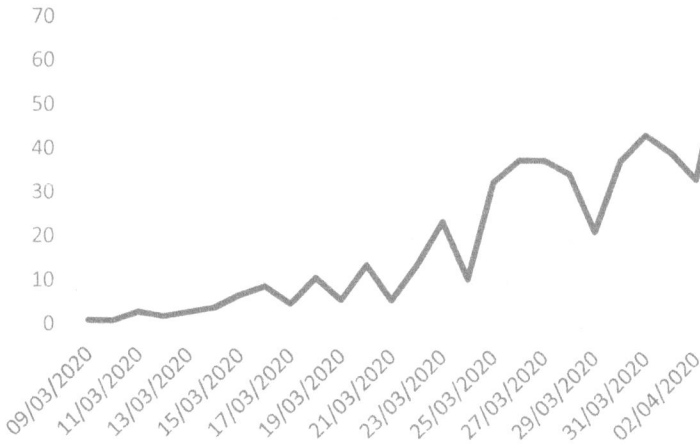

Confirmed case numbers in Newham – the First Wave.

One of our first major worries was care homes. Newham has a very young population with few very old people (in comparison to many other areas), and we also have few care homes. However, it was clear from the evidence emerging from other countries that care homes were very high-risk environments both in terms of infection spread and serious illness. Old age and underlying health conditions were already emerging from Italy as major risk factors for death from the virus. As the bed pressure on hospitals was starting to mount significantly, there was increasing pressure to have rapid discharge from hospitals of frail patients to create space for new admissions.

At times, it felt that care homes were being seen primarily by the wider system as a tool for emptying hospital beds rather than the actual homes of particularly clinically vulnerable people. But how could we safely discharge patients to care homes without knowing whether or not they were carrying Covid? How could we limit spread in our care homes without access to Personal Protective Equipment (PPE) for the staff who faced the risk of catching the virus in their daily lives and who were likely to bring Covid into the homes? It was the first issue where I felt real dissatisfaction with the system; the first moment in the pandemic when I felt confident enough that I sufficiently understood the issue to realise that the national policy was inadequate. However, the collective myopia on what was actually going on in those first few weeks of March ensured that action was simply not taken quickly enough to mitigate the risks. The tragic consequences would, once again, become apparent some weeks later.

My first real frustrations, even anger, started to emerge around these issues. While I understood that there was a shortage of tests at this early stage in the pandemic, it seemed unconscionable that people being discharged from hospital to care homes were not a priority. If testing was not going to be possible, then surely we needed to find another way?

We needed to take some control and develop local solutions. My colleague Dr Adeola Agbebiyi, a senior public health consultant in our team, who had much stronger health protection instincts, led this. Working with social care colleagues, including my ever-supportive boss Colin Ansell and others from the NHS, they developed workarounds for the absence of testing. These included agreeing, in the absence of testing, an intermediate place for the discharge of patients so we could be more confident that positive cases were not coming into our care homes, and separating potentially Covid-positive residents from others during their infectious period. This solution, alongside dedicated efforts by our care home staff to control infection spread as much as possible, would undoubtedly save many lives as the pandemic wore on, but tragically, not before lives had been lost. Not for the last time, we were needing to work out local solutions.

Throughout the pandemic, these moments of greatest frustration were brought on by a deep sense of dissonance between my sense of responsibility and my feelings of a lack of control. As a director of public health, you think and feel deeply about a place in the way, I imagine, a teacher often goes to bed thinking about their class, a doctor thinks about their patients, and I know my partner – a children's social worker – thinks about the children and families she works with. I frequently go to bed thinking about the community that I serve and the things we could do each day to protect or improve its health.

Throughout the pandemic, the knowledge that the health and wellbeing of the community we worked for was under acute threat motivated my team and me to work more hours than we had ever done before, to be innovative and creative, and to work collaboratively with people right across our community. But many times, there was stuff we couldn't do. We needed others, typically national policymakers, to make certain decisions, and that simply didn't happen. Against this background, we would use the paths available to us through official channels, such as the Association of Directors of Public Health, a tiny organisation that punched well above its weight with the government through the pandemic, or we worked with my chief executive through our local government advocacy structures.

At times, I would contact senior people in the London system with a WhatsApp or call; it was good to be able to share my experiences and feelings, even if I knew the individual impact of this advocacy was probably minimal.

I also turned to Twitter where, as the pandemic wore on, I increasingly found a place where I could connect with people in Newham to celebrate and share the good things we were doing and articulate where I felt the gaps and oversights were in the policy response. As a director of public health, like other senior officials in local government, we are – by contract – "politically restricted", highly limited in what we are allowed to say to avoid the sense that the advice we are giving local politicians is influenced by party political leanings. But we are not "policy restricted", and I always felt it was important to raise concerns around policy choices while mindful of using language that did not stray across the line. It felt helpful, even in the small echo chamber of the Twittersphere, to air my frustrations, and this would frequently lead to a call from a journalist to follow up. As one individual in one of 150 local authorities, there's no reason why anyone in particular should be heard, but Twitter definitely gave me an opportunity to amplify my voice.

As Covid started to take off locally, and as lockdown started, it was starting to become clear that the previously unimaginable was in fact very real. Indeed, almost every aspect of life was suddenly about to need to be reimagined.

Chapter 5
Gold

Many things would have been different if Covid had come ten years earlier. For example, reading Catherine Green and Sarah Gilbert's book *Vaxxers*,[9] it is striking how fortunate we were to have the benefit of ten years of progress in vaccine technology. This put us in the position where the scientific community could develop vaccines as quickly as they could. After a pandemic that began in the early months of 2020, Margaret Keenan received the first dose of what was an incredibly safe and effective range of vaccines on December 8th of the same year. That is pretty extraordinary in historical terms. Without those vaccines, it is very unclear in what timeframe we could have returned to post-pandemic normality.

There were other aspects of technology which transformed our pandemic experience, too. How would we have managed without Zoom and Teams and other new communication tools? Our work, our children's education, and our social lives would have been fundamentally different (presumably fewer quizzes!). These technologies were so central to our Covid experience.

Aside from technology, there were other significant changes. One major difference for me and my colleagues was because of the Health and Care Act 2012 (at times referred to as the Lansley reforms after Andrew Lansley, the Health Secretary who had driven the changes). This legislation moved local public health practice from being primarily based in the NHS (where I had started my public health training) back to its

---

[9] C. Green and S. Gilbert, *Vaxxers: A Pioneering Moment in Scientific History*, Hodder and Stoughton, 2022.

historic roots in local government. While there were significant concerns about aspects of the Act, I and many others thought the transition to local government for public health brought a huge opportunity. It was a move from a system (the NHS) geared towards treating illness to one that has far greater potential to improve underlying physical and mental health and to prevent poor health. Given the strength of evidence that factors such as work, housing, neighbourhoods and education are the most important determinants of health, moving to local government would shift our day-to-day working lives so much closer to those things that we thought mattered most.

It also took us from being part of the huge, centralised bureaucracy of the NHS to the much more localised world of councils. Extraordinarily, the NHS is one of the largest employers in the world (in the top ten after various armed forces, the Chinese and Indian railways, Walmart, and a couple of others). At a high level, the NHS is led by the Secretary of State, with decisions flowing down into regions and local areas in quite a strict hierarchical manner. This central direction is largely only interrupted at the level of patient care, where clinicians have professional autonomy.

Local government, by contrast, while constrained by a set of legal responsibilities and budgets which mainly come from central government, are far more autonomous and locally accountable. Councils are, in many ways, independent and guided by the decision-making of locally elected politicians with a democratic mandate and a strong sense of accountability to their communities. Despite the significant financial challenges (and maybe, in part, because of them) that local governments faced through the 2010s and into the 2020s – such as huge cuts to their budgets from central government – councils have become increasingly innovative and tried to reinvent themselves. They have also become a place where many people committed to social change come to work. As the pandemic wore on, I would find local government a place where we could be creative, driven, and with a close connection to our communities.

There is little public or (seemingly) central government awareness of the sheer scale and breadth of what councils do. This includes safeguarding and supporting vulnerable adults and children, building and providing homes, tackling homelessness, supporting schools, town planning, dealing with waste, environmental health, registering births and deaths, running elections, community safety, regeneration, parks and leisure, commissioning vital health services (like sexual health, domestic violence and substance misuse services), roads and public realm improvement, and more. Beyond those functions, lack of awareness extends to how connected local government is to its place and the communities within it (that's not to say that councils always act in this way).

By mid-March 2020, we were seriously trying to grapple with what the pandemic would mean for us as a local authority. I had been progressively briefing Althea Loderick, the chief executive, other senior directors, and Newham's mayor, Rokhsana Fiaz, plus other councillors. Increasingly, as the significance of what was happening became clear, we started to escalate our response. Existing plans, like our pandemic flu plan, provided some initial guidance, but it was apparent that systemic implications for the local authority – that would go far wider than ever anticipated – were heading our way.

There were so many unknowns and questions to answer. Which council services, that people rely on in day-to-day life, would carry on and in what way? How could a workforce of several thousand people who were not equipped for virtual work change their working practices in days and weeks rather than months and years? Who of our many frontline staff, from refuse collectors to social workers and disabled children's transport drivers, would need to carry on working in person, and how would we protect them adequately? How would we meet our responsibilities to support people living in care homes and meet the huge increase in demand to support the discharge of patients from hospital? What did it mean for schools and our support function, even though that had diminished in recent years? How would we meet the needs of our homeless population? What would be the additional responsibilities that the government or the pandemic itself would throw at us?

After several days of meetings, on March 10th, we formally declared the situation an emergency and initiated "Gold". This is the response to a major incident, as set out in the national *Emergency Response and Recovery* (non-statutory guidance), accompanying the Civil Contingencies Act of 2004, and reflected in our local plans. Gold meetings brought together all the senior directors in the council. We initially met twice a day, then daily, then a few times a week. We carried on these meetings for nearly 18 months, stopping only in the early autumn of 2021.

It would be easy to be panicked in a situation like this. As a leadership team, we were going through something none of us had encountered before; something of an all-consuming magnitude. Our chief executive, Althea Loderick, helped build a sense of focused calm. A seemingly small act of leadership by her really stayed with me. She asked a senior colleague, less directly involved with the operational response to the pandemic and an excellent meeting chair, to run the Gold meetings so she could be truly present – focused on what we were doing, not running a meeting. That lack of ego and sense of priority set an incredibly important tone.

We developed and held the ever-evolving plan, trying constantly to identify the issues our community would face and what realistically we could do to mitigate them. We worked out how to implement national policy directives as they came down and how to manage the communication challenge of the time. Local government is not typically thought of as a creative, dynamic and fast-moving environment. With the desperate need to just *get things done*, an immensely strong collective will, and some temporary loosening of some of the bureaucracy of normal local government decision-making processes (some of which are absolutely necessary to maintain democratic accountability and avoid corruption), we were able to be creative and move fast.

Among the first challenges we faced was the most basic function of any employer: how to protect our staff and those they work with. Our staff were understandably seeking clarity in a period of uncertainty and fear for some.

We were trying to follow the evidence base and emerging guidance as fast as possible while grappling with the limited information flowing down from the government, emerging scientific understanding, and our own common sense. But common sense is a hugely unreliable informant, particularly in the context of a very new challenge, which this pathogen was. For example, in those early days, we were madly wiping down surfaces while crowding into small meeting rooms. This could easily have resulted in mass infection of our senior teams as Covid spread.

I leant very heavily on my colleague, Dr Adeola Agbebiyi, in these early days and months. With a clinical background, a lot of understanding, and a highly curious and intelligent mind, she helped carve out an evidence-informed response. In the early days, we were responding to an initial trickle, then a flood of queries from schools, workplaces, and our own colleagues on how to deal specifically with symptomatic individuals. Now, we needed to provide guidance on a grand scale to handle many possible scenarios. For example, *who* should be sent home if someone had certain symptoms? What about the people who sat next to them? Who needed to come to work? If they did, how should they work in a way that maximised safety? What Personal Protective Equipment (PPE) was required by whom, what category, and how should it be worn? What cleaning regimes were needed?

PPE was a huge challenge. This acronym had probably never been used in a council senior management team meeting before, but it soon became a central topic of every Gold meeting for many weeks. There was nowhere near enough PPE in the whole system, including the NHS, and the wider system clearly needed a lot of it. But what about our services? How could we adequately protect people when personal contact was required without it?

While we were being promised PPE by central government, it was taking a while to actually arrive. One day, we were due our first much-anticipated delivery from the army. We imagined a huge army truck pitching up at the front of our offices and unloading large boxes of this precious resource that felt like gold dust. We could not believe our eyes when we saw how small the package in the lobby of our office was. We needed millions of gloves, masks and aprons to support our wider community. Crazy stories started circulating of hospitals contacting local schools to borrow safety goggles and other equipment from science labs. Was this really what was required for a health system in the sixth-largest economy in the world?[10] In a conversation with a senior doctor from the local hospital, I was asked to help find laundry services so they could get clinical scrubs cleaned as quickly as possible (this one, they managed to sort themselves).

---

[10] London hospitals appeal for masks and goggles from school science lessons, *London Evening Standard*, March 31st 2020.

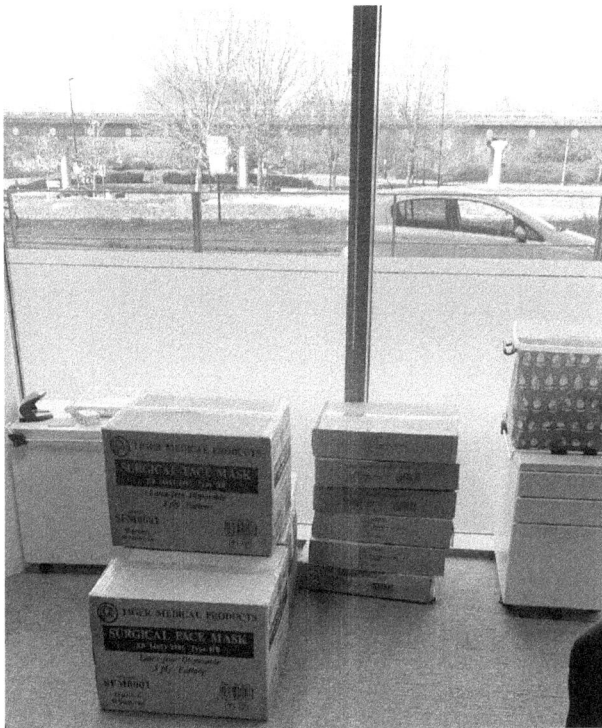

The first Army PPE delivery – we were quite surprised.

Our procurement colleagues got busy trying to source what we needed on an industrial scale. Suddenly, they were being inundated with offers from potential suppliers from all over the world. How would they determine what was authentic and high quality, and who were just chancers trying to make a fast buck out of the crisis? While the system was slowly cranking up to support the NHS, we were left to try to support the highly vulnerable social care system, our workforce, and others in the community who supported residents. I was called by the largest firm of undertakers in the borough who, sadly, were incredibly busy and unable to source PPE for their staff as they dealt with dead bodies and grieving families.

We had to set up distribution hubs – procurement, storage, and delivery – in line with the guidance to ensure PPE was used properly and efficiently (i.e., not to cause harm by misuse or waste precious resources). These highly unglamorous behind-the-scenes tasks (the kind at times derided as bureaucratic and *not frontline*) were critical in getting an effective supply chain to staff, such as care workers who needed to look after our most clinically vulnerable residents.

If the reporting of the first known Covid case in the borough was a big moment for our local colleagues and politicians, even if it was presaging a deluge, the first death was more heightened. The regular reporting of the numbers dying from Covid was a feature of the pandemic in the UK, and this was hard to take locally. As local government, we don't confront daily deaths in the same way that those working in the health service do. The deaths we know about are most typically the rarer tragic events: murders that take place which impact young people or which have a public context; domestic homicides or homelessness deaths that occur beneath the radar of local attention. However, in the context of Covid, the government published updated data on deaths for the country and each area daily.

At our Gold meetings, it was clear quite quickly that the challenge wasn't just how to communicate a small number of deaths, but more about the practical and grim task of working out what to do with the mounting number of people who were dying. Local councils have several responsibilities in this area, including the death registration process, which is required before a body can be released for burial or cremation. They are also responsible for "public health funerals" when there is no family or others to bury people (historically known as paupers' funerals).

The registration process was struggling. Firstly, there was a shortage of local authority registrars, a position that had suffered from council funding cuts. At the time, these short-staffed teams were being hit, as some staff were isolating for Covid reasons, whilst the need was rapidly escalating as fatalities mounted. There were other pressures as well. With large numbers of people dying at home, and the absence of GPs (due to a combination of workload and isolation) to certify deaths, death registration was being delayed. In addition, there was a need for greater infection control measures throughout the whole process leading up to funerals.

In areas like Newham, there were particular concerns around culturally significant practices such as ghusl, an important ritual of washing and shrouding the body in the Muslim faith. The sheer number of deaths allied to these challenges in the system was creating a backlog of funerals and a challenge on body storage capacity in London generally, and East London in particular. The existing provision simply could not cope.

As the days went on, conversations ramped up in our Gold meetings around this escalating problem. Eventually, we announced that a temporary body storage facility was to be constructed in the North East of Newham, in an area called Manor Flats; otherwise, there would be nowhere for dead bodies to be kept. It was a grim example of how our normal council conversations had gone from the idealistic at times, and often fairly mundane, to this new reality. And all in the course of a few weeks.

Planning for a makeshift body storage facility close to the neighbourhoods where people live and go about their daily lives felt almost surreal, like we were operating in a war zone. But for the residents and the local politicians, accountable and trying to lead locally, it could be quite terrifying.

Councils are political entities headed by local politicians. As much as I feel very connected to and responsible for the place where I work as DPH, our politicians are much more so. Many of our councillors grew up in Newham; all live there today and are very representative of their community, coming from many of the same ethnic and religious groups found throughout the area. They care deeply about their place and are answerable to residents at the ballot box.

Newham, in common with some councils (but still the exception rather than the norm), has a directly elected mayor: Rokhsana Fiaz. Like so many councillors, she grew up in the borough, a child of immigrant parents, and lives there to this day. One of Gold's challenges was supporting the elected members in fulfilling their leadership roles. The relationship can be complex. They rely on us for information and insight to be able to lead; they also need sufficient information and understanding to scrutinise our professional actions.

Stephen Covey writes about being able to progress in organisations "at the speed of trust" and that trust is founded on a combination of character and competence.[11] That applies closely to how I tried to foster that relationship with our local politicians and, indeed, the wider community.

As a DPH, it was vital to me that I could adequately reassure local politicians that what we were doing was the right course of action. At the same time, I was acutely aware that we were all on a huge learning curve, and we didn't know what lay around the corner. To provide reassurance, therefore, I had to build confidence in myself. The CMO meetings I mentioned earlier were vital in doing so, with the daunting expectation that I would perform a similar function locally.

Central to my approach was being 100% straightforward and honest; I didn't know the answer to every question and was unsure about many things. I had to convey that reality and show people that I was doing the right things to try to understand the situation, and that I was evidence-led in my approach. The same was true for my colleagues;

[11] S. Covey, *The 7 Habits of Highly Effective People*, Free Press, 1989.

communicating that we had a plan, being transparent about what we were doing, and being honest about uncertainty built a sense of trust. This approach, through many difficulties, would serve us well through the pandemic.

Chapter 6
HelpNewham

One week after our first confirmed Covid case, I called my (still) small team together. Sitting around the room where we regularly held normal, run-of-the-mill team meetings, I said we needed to drop pretty much everything we were doing. The day job had changed; it was all about Covid now.

Over the previous week, the debate about the need for some form of lockdown had grown much stronger. Government had made no announcements, but we were facing increasing challenges from schools and workplaces. What should head teachers, businesses, and charities do if they had people with symptoms? Who should be sent home? Who could still come to work? Indeed, how many, and on what basis? With no testing and no contact tracing in place, it wasn't totally clear what to do. What was apparent, however, was that this thing was spinning out of control and very quickly.

From the early days of Covid, I was particularly concerned not just about controlling the infection but the wider social and psychological impacts of both the epidemic and the measures that would be taken to enforce social distancing. Panic buying was widespread – notably toilet rolls (like an en-vogue Christmas toy) – and some goods were becoming scarce. With supermarkets increasingly lacking certain basic goods, my fears were compounded.

These instinctive concerns had two roots for me. My background is in the social policy and socio-economic inequalities sphere of public health rather than the medical; my first inclination was to think of poverty, hunger, and isolation, more than pathology, virus and transmission. Alongside these instincts, a more recent experience also helped shape my thinking and initial response.

Two years previously, I had been working on the recovery from the Grenfell Tower fire disaster. Like others, I had been deeply saddened by the tragedy, both by the human devastation and also the apparent failings of the state in both the cause and the immediate response. I felt a sense of shame and collective responsibility that the state, the entity I worked for, although not in that area, charged with improving people's lives, had got it so wrong. When there was an opportunity to go to North Kensington, where the disaster had happened, and try to contribute to the recovery, I wanted to be part of it. I spent nine months there trying to make sense of the disaster, not asking the questions that the public inquiry would (i.e., *why* it had occurred), but asking what – beyond the tragic death toll – the impact had been on the community, and what was needed to support their journey to recovery.

I read the disaster recovery literature widely, with research going as far back as the Aberfan colliery disaster in 1966, and more recently, the Canterbury earthquakes in New Zealand, the Lac-Mégantic train crash in Canada, 9/11, and the Enschede fireworks disaster in Eastern Netherlands. I spoke to as many people in the community as I could and looked at what data I could find. I had the privilege of being mentored by Professor Lucy Easthope, one of the UK's leading disaster experts, whose astonishing book, *When the Dust Settles*, highlights many themes of disaster response. The experience taught me many things.

Most clearly, I witnessed the complete breakdown of relationships and trust between the community and the state. The understandable anger and lack of faith in the capacity of the state to do good undermined the basic principles of democratic consent that, as a society, we rely on to govern and get stuff done. I came across a Dutch proverb dating back to 1848 that has stayed with me: *"Trust arrives on foot but leaves on horseback"*. Of course, the circumstances of the

Grenfell Tower fire disaster were extraordinary, but I ended my time there committed to trying to bridge those divides better: to build trust, to place a high value on honesty and respect, to give greater attention to the nature of race and racism in our society, and to see our communities as the most powerful assets we have for improving health and wellbeing.

The other thing I learnt about disaster situations (not just in the immediate impact, but in people's longer-term resilience) was how important the basics are – things like food, water, shelter, security, etc. – the base of Maslow's hierarchy of needs.[12] This came not just from Grenfell but was clear across the literature of the other disasters I had researched. It seems obvious, but while trying to address a disaster alongside clearing it up, attention also needs to be given to food, social isolation, medical prescriptions, employment, and children's basic needs. These aren't just basic needs in themselves, but their absence makes people much less resilient to the mental health impacts of a disaster and its consequences.

These experiences and reflections sat powerfully with me as I started to grapple with the first wave of Covid and the potential implications of lockdown. What would a lockdown mean for those lacking money and social connection, disabled people, or carers or others who relied on certain systems to manage, and which might be under threat because of prolonged social distancing? We needed to think about these issues alongside how we would manage the spread of infection.

The years leading up to the pandemic saw a shameful growth industry in the UK: the rise of food banks. When I worked in national policy around poverty earlier in my career, these were few in number. These hyper-local initiatives, almost always run by dedicated volunteers in small community or

---

[12] A. Maslow, A theory of human motivation, *Psychological Review*, 1943.

faith organisations or as part of the large Trussell Trust network, fill gaps vacated by our country's diminishing social safety net. The growth in conditionality to our benefit system, the devaluing of social security compared to the cost of living, policies like the two-child benefit limit, the wider benefit cap, complexities in the system, and – most perniciously – the new group of people with "no recourse to public funds" has left many individuals reliant on food handouts.

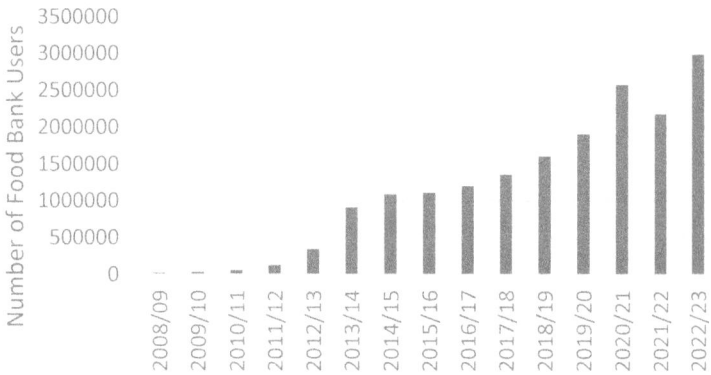

Trends in the number of users of Trussell Trust foodbanks 2008-2023. Source: UK foodbank users 2023 | Statista.

In a place like Newham, with many people living below the poverty line and a large refugee and asylum-seeking population, food bank usage was already likely to be higher than in most places. With supermarket shelves increasingly empty and queues to get in, we began to understand that access to food was going to be a real concern for a significant number of people. My colleague, Hafsa Elmi, went on a mission to find out how many active food banks there were in the borough. She found seven.

We began to think about who would need support in the next phase if, and more likely when, lockdown was announced. There had begun discussion of "shielding" – a group of people who would be required or at least strongly advised to remain at home because of the risk of serious illness if they became infected. We knew the emerging evidence and the likelihood of who may be advised to stay at home (although formal shielding advice and support had not yet been announced), and we considered those aged over 70 and living alone as likely to face particular challenges if they were advised to stay at home. Added to the mix were the barriers of language for some, digital exclusion for others, and the fact that in Newham, many would not have family nearby. The challenges seemed clear. How would some of these people get food? How would they get prescriptions? Might some feel incredibly isolated at home, with their connections to the outside world cut off?

We, of course, were not the only ones asking these questions. Alongside councils around the country, mutual aid neighbourhood WhatsApp groups were popping up. Leaflets were going through doors, inviting you to join your local group to help out with shopping for people in your community, alongside any other needs. People in their communities were starting to mobilise on a significant scale. A widely cited figure estimates that 4,300 of these "mutual aid groups" were initiated between March and May 2020[13]; an amazing community response. My colleague Phil Veasey, passionate about the role of the community, reached out across Newham and built vitally important links with many of these groups and other community organisations who were mobilising.

---

[13] A million volunteer to help NHS and others during Covid-19 outbreak | Volunteering | *The Guardian* | 13 April 2020

In Newham, however, like many population-dense urban areas, close community ties co-exist with isolation, and bottom-up community action was both vital and insufficient on its own. We needed to meet it halfway with a governmental approach, thinking about the whole population. We needed to ensure people did not fall through the cracks of our collective support efforts.

We began to design what we would call HelpNewham, a huge mobilisation of staffing and volunteers. Our ability to mobilise at scale and pace benefited from a number of key circumstances. Firstly, the council had started to downscale lots of normal operations; a vast organisation was increasingly focused on several core functions (rubbish collection and social work, for example), with many people reassigned to support the Covid response. This meant we had a large workforce we could deploy.

Secondly, from March 23rd, many people were furloughed. The unprecedented government intervention provided funds for businesses to pay people 90% of their wages not to work, ensuring that the economy didn't grind to a halt and household finances could withstand this enormous economic shock. We had already been banking on lots of volunteers to make HelpNewham work, and clearly this would make a massive difference. We had empty schools we could use as distribution hubs, and taxi drivers who would support our prescription deliveries. Finally, and equally unusually, central government had authorised local councils in the early stages of the pandemic to spend whatever was needed; the costs would be covered. We saw it as a sufficient guarantee, at that stage, to support us in being ambitious about the nature and level of help we could offer our community.

However, having a budget and a workforce alone was only the start. How do you design and mobilise a system in a number of weeks that can identify those who need support in a population of over 350,000 people and get them the assistance they need? My brilliant colleagues, led by the superpowers of Rebecca Eligon, got to work. Rebecca designed a set of work programmes, each with leads who would meet early in the morning and late in the evening each day to update on progress. There were so many complex tasks to achieve in little time. There were people focused on creating our phone bank, which would be used to call tens of thousands of residents to identify those who needed support. We didn't want to create dependency, nor did we have the resources to support those who didn't really need the help. But we also wanted to ensure that people didn't feel bad asking for help either. The challenge of Covid would leave many mostly self-sufficient people struggling, so we had to get the script right and find and train call centre staff. Walking that line was a real skill.

We needed to identify our potential target population. We agreed on risk categories, the biggest of which was people over 70 who lived alone. Even in a borough with a young population, there were thousands of people who fitted that description, and we could use our council data systems to identify those in our risk categories.

We also needed a food distribution system. What would constitute an affordable, nutritious, and – to the best extent possible – culturally-appropriate food box? How would we source and distribute it? Given that a healthy diet is one of the primary chronic public health challenges of our time, we fortunately had people in the team who knew what they were doing. Racha Fayad, a nutritionist, could advise on box contents, and the indefatigable Andy Gold, our head of food strategy, had worked in industry and knew about supply and distribution. We needed to work with the pharmacies in the area, too, in order to help get prescriptions to isolating residents. We designed a volunteer befriending service so that people who felt lonely could have someone checking in for a chat. We also needed infection control to ensure that while trying to help our local population, we minimised the risk of spreading Covid and inadvertently doing more harm than good. Behind all this, we needed logistics to make sure everything worked, from food deliveries and packaging to volunteer recruitment training and management.

It wasn't all about direct delivery, either. We knew that many people would seek help not from the council but from a local community organisation: a mosque, church, or local community centre. We began to support small grassroots voluntary and community and faith organisations already reaching out to others in the community.

Many people will be familiar with the food bank model, providing cans of tinned tuna, custard, pasta, and rice… all non-perishables. But what about fresh food? Fruit, vegetables, meat, and fish? There was a substantial new surplus from London's catering industry – how could we ensure it didn't go to waste? We provided commercial fridges to countless small community organisations, plus training on food safety, so we could include fresh food in our distribution and provide rounded diets to people.

As a council, we mobilised this response in a matter of weeks. It was driven by a team that was incredibly ambitious and innovative in trying to support the residents of our area.

April 2nd 2020, Curwen Primary School, Plaistow

A few days into the start of our HelpNewham operation, I went to Curwen Primary School in Plaistow to see the set-up and meet some of the staff and volunteers who had facilitated this extraordinary response. There, I was met by Syed Haque. In previous roles, Syed had overseen humanitarian responses overseas as well as army logistics. These days, he worked as a Head of a community centre and library in Newham. We couldn't have been luckier. Day and night, Syed worked to build a food distribution system on the ground that worked like a military operation but with infection control. I was completely in awe of what he and others had achieved. After visiting the site and chatting with the staff and volunteers, the mayor was due to come to do the same. I was waiting on the drive to the school as she arrived, and when I saw her, I burst into tears. It was incredibly uncharacteristic; I don't think I have ever cried before at work. But it was an outpouring of pent-up anxiety and stress from one of the most intense months of my life. Looking back, I can't really believe that we were only really one month into the pandemic; in reality, it had only just begun.

By the time we closed down HelpNewham in August 2020 (evolving it into more sustainable approaches to community support), over 30,000 residents had been contacted to identify if they needed help (nearly 10% of the population), 80,000 food parcels had been delivered supporting 7,800 families, 15,000 prescriptions were delivered, and over 3,200 family boxes were provided. Thanks to the work of Sally Burns, our public mental health lead, a new befriending scheme was launched, too, reaching nearly 1,000 isolated residents in need of support.

As one resident said, *"We were so grateful; we would never have got through it otherwise. They always came on time, they always had a chat, they were so nice... We are in our late 70s; without this service, we would have been stumped."*[14]

Today, from the seven food banks Hafsa identified in March 2020, there are now more than 35 food banks or other kinds of community and faith groups delivering surplus food in the borough. The challenge changed as the pandemic evolved and then we transitioned into a cost-of-living crisis; significant need grew and endured. On the one hand, the

---

[14] Learning From HelpNewham (2020), a Report by Social Engine.

growth of food banks is a source of positive community mobilisation, but equally shameful is the weakness of our safety nets in such an affluent society.

We also learned a lot from the experience about the state's role in providing support. Two things particularly stand out to me about how we support individuals and how we work with community.

So often, the relationship between the state and those seeking support is transactional. It is an evolved response to try to simplify complexity and make limited budgets stretch in a legally justifiable way. Whether people need support around social care, housing, income, or special educational needs for their children, we define categories narrowly and strictly, we assess people to see if they qualify to fit in any boxes, we rule them out or in, and then if they hit some threshold (often defined in law), they get a specific kind of support. With HelpNewham, we were uncharacteristically open. Were people concerned? Did they have support from family, friends, or others in the community? What were they most concerned about? We tried to build connections based on empathy and trust and used that as a basis for finding the right kind of support, which wasn't always a "service". It created a very different kind of relationship between our staff and residents that we would build on later in the pandemic.

In terms of community, we increasingly saw ourselves not just as "doers" but "enablers". There is a "statist" view of the world which – at its extreme – says if there is an important need to be met in the community, then government should try to meet it. If we spent £1 million on buying food and delivering it directly to people, we could reach a certain number of people; in turn, we would have a large level of control over that intervention and see very clearly the impact of our work. But if we made common cause with our community, and we spent that £1 million to develop the community infrastructure (from fridges to volunteer support), we could reach far more people, including those who would *not* come to the state to seek help for all kinds of reasons. HelpNewham was successful because it evolved on that basis, and over time, we increasingly "did" less and "enabled" more. This partnership between local government and community – around a sense of common purpose – would be something we would continue to build on.

Chapter 7
Same Storm, Different Boats

The slow, slow, then fast experience of Covid came a couple of weeks later to our hospitals. At first, there was an initial drip of patients, but a flood quickly followed. London's hospitals were suddenly under enormous pressure, with very unwell people coming into Emergency Departments in huge numbers and many needing intensive care.

The sheer numbers coming through placed incredible demands on hospital staff as Covid was a new illness, with little evidence base or understanding of how best to treat it. Clinicians were working things out on the hoof, using their judgement, and sharing WhatsApp messages with other doctors from other hospitals here and overseas, where they had been seeing Covid for a little bit longer. Medics would read whatever they could find from colleagues when they got home at night, exhausted.

The challenge was made harder by immediate large staff absences, either because people were symptomatic, unwell, or shielding because of personal risk conditions.

Vital clinical tools were under great pressure, too, in particular ventilators and oxygen to help support people's breathing. The situation required two TV hospital dramas, *Casualty* and *Holby City*, to donate their actual ventilators to the real-life cause (enough to make you wonder about global healthcare inequalities, which this book will touch on briefly towards the end).

Bedspace was filling up so quickly that it was unclear whether London would cope. The hospitals were frantically creating more intensive care capacity where they could, repurposing other wards and operating theatres to be able to take more ventilated patients. As fast as they were creating new capacity, intensive treatment units were filling up, and with no confidence in where the peak of cases would be, there was concern that the existing hospital infrastructure would reach its absolute limit. I would get daily updates from our local hospital, Newham University Hospital, sometimes exchanging messages just to check on colleagues – like the medical director's wellbeing – and sometimes making a phone call if I felt I needed a bit more information. The calls were becoming increasingly despairing.

No one wanted to be in the position we had seen in Italy, where corridors were full of ill patients, and awful rationing decisions were being made about which patients would be prioritised for care. Indeed, in late March 2020, I was asked to join an ethics panel with hospital doctors in North East London to start considering these unthinkable questions. How would we ration access to different aspects of critical care, if and when the time came?

Having run out of available space in existing hospitals, the NHS responded to this challenge by building a field hospital: a makeshift site that could take thousands of extra patients. I received an early phone call (mostly as a welcome courtesy, as it was on my patch) to say the cavernous Excel Exhibition Centre was being considered as the potential site.

Over a couple of days, senior officials in the NHS debated matters and worked out what might be possible, and then – in just a few more days, with the help of the Army – they put together what would be the first Nightingale Hospital. The Excel Centre, five minutes' walk from my office in Newham, typically hosts the London triathlon, countless trade fairs, and is normally full in early April with runners coming to register for the London marathon. However, this year, there would be no marathon runners, just doctors, nurses, and the others needed to make a hospital function.

The facility's opening understandably caused anxiety for some of our residents. Was our situation so bad that we needed an emergency hospital in Newham? In truth, it was a facility for all of London and even wider. By the time it was complete and ready to open, we hoped the epidemic's peak had passed, and it would not see too many patients. In all likelihood, had it been fully required, it would have been an enormous challenge for the health system. It is one thing to build a field hospital in this kind of emergency situation; it is a wholly different challenge to adequately staff it when all the existing hospitals in the system are struggling to staff sufficient doctors and nurses.

Planned for thousands of patients at its peak, the Nightingale Hospital in the end had just 57 admissions. As a King's Fund report has suggested, looking back at the emergency, makeshift Nightingale Hospitals could either be seen as *"White elephants that could never have been used, or as the ultimate insurance policy that were thankfully not needed."*[15]

April 2020

On April 5th, the UK's Prime Minister, Boris Johnson, was admitted to Guy's and St Thomas' Hospital, located on just the other side of Westminster Bridge from the Houses of Parliament. Initially, the noises coming out of 10 Downing Street were that this was purely precautionary, but as the next couple of days wore on, it became clear his situation was serious. On April 7th, he was moved to an Intensive Treatment Unit (ITU). For a few days, much of the country was focused on this situation; it seemed unthinkable that a Prime Minister could die in office in a pandemic. As news of his recovery subsequently seeped out, the country – political divisions put to one side – breathed a collective sigh of relief,

---

[15] The King's Fund, *Was Building the NHS Nightingale Hospitals Worth the Money?* May 2021

and on April 12th, he was out of the danger zone and discharged to recover at home.

For those few days, the Prime Minister's predicament reinforced a feeling that existed in the early days of the pandemic. Namely, that we were all in this together, equally impacted by this cruel virus. If the virus could get to the Prime Minister, none of us were safe. Of course, that was true to some degree, but soon it became clear that the risks for some people were lower than for others.

It seems obvious with hindsight (it often does), but those of us watching most closely had only just started to think about potential ways in which social factors might be having an impact on individuals who were most at risk.

The first indicator for me was a Tweet I saw on April 3rd, tracking the pandemic in its early days in the US.

"The #Covid19 death rate highest in metro Albany GA, New Orleans, New York, and Detroit. Death rates higher in colder, wetter, denser places – and with higher Black, Asian and Hispanic share." (Tweet from Jed Kolko, April 3rd 2020)[16]

It made me reflect on our own area. What would be the causal mechanisms operating that meant people from minority groups could have disproportionately higher mortality rates from Covid? At this point, still so early in the global pandemic, there was very little published data (some data had started to emerge in the UK from a national audit of critical care), and it was too soon for peer-reviewed journals; Twitter would have to do.

One thing we knew with confidence, at this point, was that old age was the number one risk factor. Aside from whether someone has been vaccinated, that remains true today. However, if there existed higher risks in minority populations

---

[16] https://twitter.com/jedkolko/status/1246157538988421120?s=21

in the US, might there be similar patterns of mortality in the UK?

At that stage, there was little granular data to understand patterns in the UK, let alone at a more local level. From a mortality perspective, it was still extremely early in the first wave. In fact, five days after having seen that tweet (i.e., April 8th), we would witness the day with the most recorded deaths in the first wave in the UK: 1,073. There was still a long wait before Wave 1 was complete. In turn, it would take sophisticated analysis, looking at multiple factors and comparing different geographical areas, to truly understand the risks associated with mortality.

However, I began to think there may be good reason to believe similar patterns could emerge in the UK, and for me, given Newham's population, that was a worry. I spent a few days reading more and thinking about it, and on April 8th, I shared a note I had written with senior colleagues. It was entitled *Newham and risk factors for COVID-19 mortality*.

There were two aspects of risk that I was trying to understand at that stage:

1. The risks of being infected (irrespective of whether that infection caused severe disease or no symptoms at all).

2. The risks of severe/fatal illness for those who had caught Covid-19.

In previous chapters, I discussed the factors that may have put Newham's residents at a greater risk of infection. In terms of the chance of becoming infected, first of all there was the sheer bad luck of living in London, where Covid took root initially. But what concerned me most were those wider determinants of health – the socioeconomic factors of jobs, housing, density, transport and community connection were all likely to put people at greater risk of catching Covid in the first place.

But what about severe and fatal illness? Again, there was a range of risk factors. There was good evidence from China that underlying health conditions had increased mortality risk. This evidence had helped inform the government's shielding advice for people with a range of conditions, particularly heart disease and diabetes. As discussed earlier, the combination of low income and ethnicity means there are very high rates of such conditions in Newham. In turn, there were linked risk factors that seemed to emerge from the evidence base (for example, smoking and obesity), which all seemed to increase people's risk.

There were more potential risk factors, too. For example, we began to consider the potential risk associated with multi-generational living. Like community life, here was something rooted in positive choice – how to support older family members, and how to cope financially where property prices are high – but which carried additional risk in certain circumstances.

In Newham, especially among certain migrant communities, it is far more common for adult children to have their parents living with them. Forty percent of those aged over 70 in Newham live with someone else of working age (compared to fewer than 10% in many places). If those younger adults were spending their days out in the community, facing the risk factors of work, population density, transport, and then bringing the virus back to their elderly relatives, that could increase the risk for those people compared to those who lived alone.

In addition, what about timely access to healthcare? We knew the language and cultural barriers that many in our community faced. It has long been recognised that despite the NHS's universality and being largely free at the point of delivery, access to care is often constrained, with sharp elbows and cultural capital helping some to gain help quicker. What if some in our community had struggled disproportionately to access medical help or advice in a timely way? Something that seemed particularly likely when the services were under such acute pressure. What about if some people took to heart the government's message, repeated every night at the Prime Minister and CMO's press conferences, to "stay at home, protect the NHS" and sought medical help too late? These factors are incredibly hard to evidence, but talking to colleagues working in Emergency Departments, they felt there was a high likelihood that this was a factor for some.

As the pandemic progressed, we could now see the number of deaths for each local authority in the country, published each day by the government. But, early on, it wasn't straightforward to compare one area with another, and it would be easy to draw the wrong conclusions. The main drivers in terms of absolute mortality, the total number of people dying, were likely to be:

- Where in the cycle of the epidemic a geographical place was. Those in London had been hit first, so death rates were likely to be higher there, but that wouldn't necessarily hold as the epidemic spread.

- Those with larger populations. The numbers here were easier to quantify with readily available statistics, although they were not necessarily accounted for in all commentary.

- Those with an older population profile, given the primary vulnerability related to age.

It would require a certain amount of data from the first extended period of the pandemic and robust statistical analyses to understand what else might be going on, and rather than absolute mortality, the relative risk of mortality that different parts of the population were exposed to.

May 2020

On the first Friday of May 2020, not much more than one month after the first national lockdown and through the whirlwind of the first extraordinary period of the pandemic, the UK's Office for National Statistics published age-standardised mortality rates for every local authority in England from Covid-19.[17] This was still very early in the pandemic, so the analysis was based on around 90,000 deaths at this point. These rates did not account for the "London" effect of where the pandemic had first taken root. What was evident in the data was that the 11 areas with the highest mortality rates at this point were all London local authorities. Other than that, it was the first major analysis that compared death rates in different places, accounting for the different sizes and age profiles of different populations. In a nutshell, we now had information on which places had the highest death rates.

Newham came top of the list. The differences between areas at this point were staggering. As the table below shows, many parts of the UK – including many more rural areas – were comparatively spared by Covid at this point, at least in terms of measured mortality.

---

[17] Deaths involving COVID-19 by local area and socioeconomic deprivation - Office for National Statistics (ons.gov.uk)

Highest 10	
Newham	144.3
Brent	141.5
Hackney	127.4
Tower Hamlets	122.9
Haringey	119.3
Harrow	114.7
Southwark	108.1
Lewisham	106.4
Lambeth	104.3
Ealing	103.2
Lowest 10	
Norwich	2.5
West Lindsey	3.6
South Hams	4.0
East Devon	4.8
Ceredigion	5.4
Somerset West & Taunton	5.5
Mendip	5.9
Mid Devon	5.9
East Lindsey	6.3
Hastings	6.4

Table: Standardised mortality rates by local area from Covid 19, March 1 to April 17 2020; ten areas with the highest and lowest standardised mortality rates.

As the news sunk in, I felt despondent. The area I felt responsible for was top of a list where no one would ever want to be. On the one hand, you tell yourself "demography is destiny", and the primacy of London, Marmot's social determinants of health, underlying inequalities, and the range of risk factors made the place a sitting duck. On the other hand, I believe my job is purposeful, that we can bend the arc of inevitability and improve people's circumstances. Otherwise, what is the point? That's what had motivated me to work in Newham in the first place.

The report had come out on a Friday, and when I woke up the next morning, I tweeted:

"Trying to reflect on the reality that Newham, where I work as Director of Public Health, has been hardest hit, along with other parts of London, by Covid-19 - the data is shocking and sobering but unsurprising too - we knew our communities face a lot of risk."[18]

I then reiterated the accumulated evidence on risk and concluded:

"There aren't easy fixes here – the challenges both to exposure and severity are deep but this data makes us more and more determined to do what we can as my brilliant colleague @rebeccaeeligon who has done so much in this response has said "tired, angry but inspired" – that's about right."

I received lots of supportive comments. That weekend, unusually, I spent time on the phone with Rokhsana and Althea, the mayor of Newham and chief executive of the council, respectively. Over the previous two months, I had grown closer to both as my role had taken on far greater prominence in council life. We spoke regularly, snatching five minutes whenever we could to work through a particular challenge, as well as all the time we spent in meetings with other senior council officers, politicians and the wider

---

[18] https://twitter.com/strelitz_jason/status/1256468774334717952

community. We all felt similarly. We felt proud of many aspects of our response over the previous two months, including the huge mobilisation around HelpNewham, Care Homes, PPE provision, and supporting council staff. We also weren't naïve as to the powers and tools at our disposal, but as people with a huge sense of responsibility to the borough in our different roles, it was devastating.

At the same time, we were collectively resolved. We didn't know how the pandemic would play out from this point on – no one did – but we agreed we didn't want to have any regrets. Anything meaningful that we could do to protect and support our community, we would try to do.

The first wave in London had subsided for now, although we were only just starting to realise that. But we were convinced that the end was a long way away, and we had time to think things through. Given the risks in our community, we knew we needed to do more.

Chapter 8
Flying Blind

For months, we simply did not know where our Covid cases were. Since the very earliest days of the pandemic – when directors of public health would get alert calls around individual cases – we only received daily emails of anonymous cases with incomplete postcodes, notifying us of positive Covid infections in our borough. We didn't even get proper details of cases in our care homes. Choose your idiom or cliché, "flying blind", "working with one hand tied behind your back" – that is how it felt.

Here we were, desperate to try to protect our communities, wanting to marshal the available resources of local authorities, volunteers, and community groups towards that shared goal, and simply unable to do many of the things our training and our experience taught us we should be doing. As directors of public health, we had been trained in health protection, the management of infectious diseases. We could see a system that was not able to cope (and missing opportunities), but were not being given the basic tools to do our job.

Through the pandemic, there was a lot of focus on R_0, the basic reproduction number. Where R_0, is above 1, every infected individual passes the virus on to, *on average*, more than 1 other person. In that situation, therefore, across a population, the number of those infected rise. Where R_0 is below 1, each infected individual, *on average*, transmits the virus to fewer than 1 person, and the overall number of cases falls.

R_0 is influenced by different things. Firstly, different pathogens have different levels of infectivity. So, measles and chickenpox have high basic reproduction numbers – a single person infected will (on average) pass those infections on to a relatively high number of people – while the influenza virus is much lower. With no other constraints, measles and chickenpox will spread much more quickly. But R_0 is then influenced by a range of factors that may support infection spread or limit it.

With greater knowledge of where confirmed cases of Covid were in our communities, we would be able to do different things that could potentially break the chains of the infection's transmission from one person to another and keep R_0 either nearer to or below 1. Without the information, we were missing some of our most powerful tools to act.

If we knew who had tested positive for Covid in our area, we could try to support the individuals not to spread the infection any further, ensuring they understood the risks. We could try to identify those who were most likely to have caught the virus from them (e.g., people they live with, close friends and colleagues), by using what is termed contact tracing. We could then try to limit the onward spread to others. This information also helped us identify specific locations where transmission was occurring – for example, a shop, a business, or a place of worship – and work with that place to try to limit any further spread.

For months and months, we were unable to do any of this due to the anonymous case and part-postcode emails.

This lack of information was hugely frustrating. The withholding of data from us was not the result of technical system problems that needed to be solved so that the data could be shared. That would have been exasperating but understandable. No, in the early months of the pandemic, it was a purposeful decision. We were being told, "This is on a need-to-know basis, and you don't need to know."

But before going into the detail, it's worth taking a step back and touching on quite how important "data" is and how it is perceived in the public health arsenal; it's sometimes close to a religion.

Since John Snow's seminal moment in the slums of Soho and Chadwick's surveys, discussed in Chapter 1, data has been so central to the public health methodology that – as a profession – we are sometimes mocked for our obsession with it and accused of "paralysis by analysis". Indeed, there are times when public health as a discipline can be so immersed in trying to understand a problem that we don't get around to actually trying to deal with it.

The focus on data can manifest in different ways. At a policy level, it leads to a committed focus on using "evidence-based" interventions; in other words, doing things that there is good reason to think will actually work. This may sound obvious, but common-sense notions of what works in medicine and social policy have repeatedly been shown to make significant mistakes.

In public health, there is a strong commitment to a hierarchy of evidence with a particular focus on the so-called "truth test" – the randomised controlled trial. The RCT was a hugely important scientific breakthrough that tackled the hardest question in interventional research: How do you know that action x has caused outcome y? Other research methods can indicate possible links between variables and outcomes, generating hypotheses that need further scrutiny, but RCTs are seen as essential to evaluations in a range of areas, including drug trials, medical and psychological treatments, and social interventions. They are considered the "gold standard" of intervention research, and a systematic review or meta-analysis of multiple high-quality RCTs, focusing on the same question, is widely considered the best possible evidence for identifying a causal relationship between an intervention and an outcome.

RCTs are a less straightforward tool in uncontrolled settings or when the intervention is more complex than the delivery of an uncomplicated, replicable intervention, like a drug. The long-running debate about the relative effectiveness of face coverings during the Covid pandemic ran up against this tension.

Beyond the particular qualities of RCTs, there are many forms of data – both quantitative and qualitative – that are equally vital in informing public health action.

At a local public health level, data is used to drive local action – whether by health services, local government, or others – to not only do what is most likely to make a positive difference but also to utilise limited resources where they are most needed. We routinely produce what we call "needs assessments", an analysis of a particular issue, which could be anything from child mental health to dementia. What is the size and nature of the issue locally? What are we doing to address it? Where are the gaps? What does the evidence suggest we should be doing differently? These questions are absolutely core to the public health method, and a reasonable level of data literacy is a prerequisite for being a qualified public health practitioner.

So, data is critical to our sense of how we do our job as public health professionals, and we didn't have it. The way I understood it, there were three very different things going on that justified the lack of data we were receiving to help us manage the pandemic locally. The first was the focus on developing NHS Test and Trace, the infamously monikered "world-class" nationally organised operation for contact tracing. The second aspect was a very particular view of data protection rules and our roles in local government. The third was linked to this and reflected fragmentation in the public health system.

NHS Test and Trace has received plenty of commentary and analysis already, which I won't repeat here. Looking back, there was a legitimate view that the scale of the challenge and mobilisation required a national approach. There is some sense in the notion that when building a large operational response that requires data systems, recruitment, and protocols, you should do things once rather than 150 times in each local authority around the country.

So, while legitimate from my perspective, I and many others thought Test and Trace was limited and ignored the benefits of collaboration as well as the mobilisation capabilities and different skills within local government. When NHS Test and Trace was eventually launched at the end of May 2020, it would clearly have systems and the scale required for a vast national approach. What it lacked, though, was speed, agility, local knowledge and relationships.

I will talk later about the barriers surrounding isolation that many people in Newham's communities and elsewhere around the country experienced, but from the beginning of the debate around contact tracing, it seemed obvious that a remote national call centre would face some particular challenges in multicultural areas. Phoning people up cold, asking very personal questions, and making profound requests of people's behaviour is not a straightforward action with predictable results. It requires empathy and the building of trust; it may also need language skills and even local knowledge to truly support some people.

While the challenge of local authority mobilisation around contact tracing would have been considerable, ignoring local authorities left us, as directors of public health, out of the picture and appeared to ignore the presence and expertise of our environmental health officer colleagues.

As mentioned earlier, environmental health officers emerged with the birth of organised public health in the mid-1840s, and they are a core part of local government life. In contemporary local government life, they still play a largely unknown role in reducing the risk of spreading infectious diseases. In pre-pandemic times, when there were outbreaks of food poisoning, potential blood-borne viruses (such as hepatitis B linked to community settings), or a viral environmental hazard such as legionella, the public health authorities (most recently Public Health England) would contact environmental health officers (EHOs) to do the legwork on the ground. They would be the ones going out and about, cold-calling strangers, knocking on doors to ask often deeply personal questions, and getting intrusive questionnaires filled in. They were the ones responsible for contact tracing to find others potentially at risk of harm or spreading disease, as well as trying to identify settings at risk.

Put another way, this existing workforce – already employed in local government – knew what they were doing. Later in the pandemic, when we started to receive data and started to build a local response, our deeply knowledgeable, experienced and thoughtful EHOs like Kerry Wood and Bill Adolph would be absolutely invaluable. For now, though, that experience was simply ignored. Other NHS-based professionals with significant experience in contact tracing, such as sexual health advisors and tuberculosis nurses, were also left out of the picture until local contact tracing efforts began.

Another factor that blocked local action from very early on was concern about what would be the legal and legitimate use of people's personal data. Again, I understood where the reasoning stemmed from, but I thought it completely wrong. Most people have some concerns about how their personal data is used, and probably no more so than when it comes to our health. We give information about ourselves for one purpose, and do not want it to be shared against our knowledge with others for other reasons (although most of us use the internet routinely in ways that suggest we don't actually mind that much!). Data protection rules have been developed to try to provide a legal architecture that protects our concerns.

It was either a combination of genuine legal concerns or the perceived spirit of the law that stopped this information from being shared. For weeks, in the early days of the pandemic, I would beg for more information. My argument was quite clear that there was a straightforward health benefit to the public for the information to be shared. We were knocked back when told that this simply wasn't our responsibility. Truthfully, I found it incredible. I would go to bed worrying about protecting my community, only to be told the next day that I couldn't have individual data because that wasn't my responsibility.

In a sense, both of these factors were bolstered by a third: the instinct that different bits of the system should "stay in their lane" and do their job and not interfere with others. It's a deeply damaging instinct that can be seen in the worst of all kinds of public services. In contrast, the best public services see deep collaboration as the best answer to the complex challenges we face in society. How do you solve difficult challenges like youth violence, social isolation, or health-based unemployment if each bit of the system – whether schools, the NHS, councils, or employment services – just "stay in their lane" without trying to cooperate on these shared problems? Here we were, grappling with a new virus, and trying to do what we thought was necessary, but essentially being told not to worry because other bits of the system would manage. They couldn't.

Eventually, in late July 2020, after lots of advocacy by people much more senior than me, and debate in government, we started to receive the data. A daily updated listing of every person in our area who tested positive for Covid. The data included their name, age, gender, address, when they had the test, the type of test, and sometimes ethnicity or occupation, proving that it could have been shared all along.

For us, it was transformative.

At last, five months into the pandemic, we were able to build a much stronger picture of where infections were in our community and try to tackle risk. But we could go further than that. Now that we knew which people had Covid, we could try to mitigate some of the limitations of the NHS Test and Trace system. Test and Trace had successfully been created at an enormous scale and was having some success in reaching our population, but its limitations – in terms of really understanding our communities and how to support them – continued to concern us. Without ever wanting to duplicate resources or annoy our residents with even more phone calls from a contact tracing system, we needed to try to work out how we could make the "world-class" system a little bit closer to what we thought was needed to support our residents. I pick this up in Chapter 12.

Chapter 9
Black Lives Matter

On May 25th 2020, George Floyd, a 46-year-old African American man, was murdered by a police officer in Minneapolis as he faced the floor, handcuffed, with the police officer's knee on his neck. The following day, footage of the incident, taken by Darnella Frazier, a 17-year-old passerby on her phone, spread across the world, sparking a wave of protests. George Floyd's words as he was held down, *"I can't breathe"*, were particularly poignant when it was clear – at that point – that so many Black and Asian people had died of Covid, a respiratory virus that left people literally breathless.

On May 31st 2020, the first large demonstrations took place around the UK to protest George Floyd's murder and the broader issues of police killings and institutional racism. At that moment, the long-standing narrative that this was just a problem in gun-saturated US society had been punctured. The protests were not just about solidarity, with events across the pond, but similar issues faced by the Black population in the UK, including examples of police shootings here, deaths in custody, being stopped for the crime of "driving while being Black", and concern over the treatment of Black victims of crime. All of this allied to wider experiences of racism and racial injustice.

Some were concerned about these demonstrations as potential Covid super spreader events. I obviously hoped they would not be, but I believed that these issues were of great importance and that people's voices needed to be heard. It helped that, in London particularly, there was little Covid around at that time, and we thought, correctly, being outdoors was much safer still in limiting the spread of infections.

The emerging evidence on the disproportionate, unequal burden of Covid that was being experienced by Black and Asian communities was a cause for deep soul searching. For a period of time, it seemed to feature regularly on the news, with statements of concern by politicians. There was the narrative that I would hear, even in multi-ethnic Newham, that the disproportionate death rate among these communities was because people weren't respecting the rules and were, therefore, at least partly to blame. This was clearly nonsense and racist. The high death rates of the first wave in London had largely been down to infections that spread before any rules were even in place. Not long after lockdown started, we reached the peak of transmission in London; it was clear that the vast majority of people were following the rules. There had to be other things that would explain what was happening.

A study was commissioned by Public Health England and led by the brilliant Professor Kevin Fenton,[19] the lead for public health in London (a friend and inspiring mentor to me and many others, I should add), to understand better what had occurred. I could see in my data that people in our borough, and particularly those of South Asian, Black Caribbean, or Black African heritage, had died at younger average ages compared to the wider population across the country as a whole. Professor Fenton's report confirmed that.

Historically, the prevailing discourse on health inequalities in the UK has predominantly been colour-blind and typically focused on socio-economic inequalities. However, the clarity of this data meant that the ethnic and racial dimension of inequalities could no longer be subsumed into a discourse

---

[19] K. Fenton, *Understanding the Impact of Covid-19 on BAME Groups*, Public Health England, 2020.

solely focused on socio-economic factors and class. What was it about the experience of race and racism that may have contributed to these premature deaths?

By the end of May 2020, we were clearly past the first wave in London. Hospital admissions and deaths had reduced to very small numbers, and the enduring lockdown conditions were keeping the virus at bay. That was not true all over the country where the virus had arrived later. In places such as Leicester, Liverpool, and Leeds, the gradual opening up that was taking place seemed to allow the virus to remain sufficiently in circulation to keep the number of infections high. Although things were looking much better in London, we knew a second wave was highly likely.

All the evidence suggested that, in the absence of vaccination, as society opened up more, there were likely to be more cases, and we assumed it might happen in the autumn as the colder weather began again. Whilst it was difficult to estimate the number who had caught Covid in the first wave, we estimated that a very small proportion of the population had been infected.

The context gave us some time but also a sense of urgency.

Disentangling the relative impacts of "race" and "socio-economic" factors is complex and a job for academic research. Clearly, of course, the two are connected; the experience of racism is itself a contributor to socio-economic disadvantage because of people's experience in education and employment that so profoundly shape people's economic trajectories.

Our focus needed to be more practical, drawing on the existing evidence. What could we do that might make a difference? Naturally, we knew that the prevalence of long-term conditions, such as diabetes, was an issue, particularly impacting our Black and Asian communities, and the wider evidence of health inequalities was obvious. There were other anecdotal reports about barriers in terms of access to care, and although some of these were hard to evidence, the impact needed to be assessed.

As we reflected on the disproportionate effect of the pandemic on Black and Asian populations, we asked two sets of questions. The first looked at the short term. Were there things we could do to protect people better in a second wave? It had been hugely disturbing to hear about people working in the NHS or social care who said they were denied PPE because of their social position or felt unable to ask, people taking on duties that they felt powerless to refuse, or concerns that some had not accessed care quickly enough because of a lack of confidence and the sharp elbows that are sometimes required.

I spoke with my colleagues in Newham's Emergency Department, who had faced such enormous challenges in the first wave. It was hard to quantify, but they worried deeply that some residents had sought medical help far too late for preventable reasons. So, if there were things we could do in preparation for a second wave, I felt it was vital that we tried.

However, we also wanted to ask a longer-term question: what could we do about the longstanding issues of racism and racial injustice? Whilst we were realistic about our ability to mitigate risk in the short term, these are not challenges with straightforward solutions. It is hard to understand the primary causes of unequal outcomes in the first place, let alone effectively implement solutions that would quickly make a difference. Indeed, many of the challenges are rooted in centuries of racism and oppression and accumulated generational and lifetime disadvantages. Given that, could we use this moment of reflection, heightened by the Black Lives Matter movement, as a catalyst for addressing longer-standing issues of disadvantage? As Albert Einstein said famously, *"In the midst of every crisis lies great opportunity."*

To respond effectively, we needed to be talking to our communities. It does no good for professionals just to sit in offices (or, in this case, on Zoom chats) deciding what is best for our population. We bring a range of expertise – an understanding of the evidence base, specialist knowledge in specific areas, an understanding of the levers of change and how to get certain things done – but these perspectives have to be allied to those of our residents and what we often refer to as their "lived experience". Without that, our understanding is limited.

Only with community knowledge and insight can broader professional expertise be meaningfully applied to context. But it goes further. Talking to communities creates a partnership, a sense that the relationship between state and citizen is not one of those with power "doing to" but of a sense of "working with", through a shared challenge.

We began talking with professionals from different disciplines, and establishing different forums for speaking to our community. We already had a very active faith network, talking to representatives from many communities in the borough. We had relationships with our voluntary and community organisations. By their very nature, in a population of over 70% of people from Black and Asian backgrounds, these groups had significant reach into our diverse communities. We established a specific reference group and invited community members to join. In addition, we had our Covid Health Champions, whom I will talk about in the next chapter.

Over time, we would increasingly look at many issues through this lens. In terms of short-term issues, however, there were certain things that particularly concerned us.

As discussed earlier, the initial phase of the pandemic had extremely limited testing. The government then committed to a significant expansion in community testing so that anyone with symptoms could get a PCR test. Drive-through test sites had been operating since the end of April in the car parks of Ikea shopping centres and other venues; for Newham's residents, the O2 entertainment complex in Greenwich was the nearest site. Gradually, the eligibility for these sites increased.

Two months later, these were still largely the only places where you could get a test unless you were admitted to hospital. However, half of our population did not have access to a car. How could we have a system in place for something so important that excluded half our population? It's a primary example of the "Inverse Care Law" coined by GP Dr Julian Tudor Hart, 50 years ago.[20] This is the principle that the availability of good medical care is often inversely correlated with the population's needs; put simply, the poorest get the worst care.

Towards the end of June, we began discussions with the Department of Health and Social Care about opening up one of the first walk-in sites in the country. In truth, we were still nervous about infection control issues at these walk-in venues. Our understanding of the relative risk of catching Covid in different contexts was still fairly limited at this stage, but we thought it was vital to create these facilities for our residents.

We also tried to work with our GPs to create access to tests for those who we thought would face barriers to testing. This was one of our projects that we never successfully launched. It remains an oddity, throughout the pandemic, that GPs and primary care more broadly – the lynchpins of our approach to diagnosis in the British healthcare system – were largely sidelined from Covid diagnosis. People were tested individually in private and then tried to seek help when their symptoms got worse. That probably worked for many but

---

[20] J. Tudor The inverse care law, *Lancet*, 1971

left some, particularly more vulnerable residents, exposed because they were not getting the support and guidance around seeking help that would happen in normal times.

As mentioned earlier, along with these challenges around testing, we were equally concerned with the trace systems. How effective would the national test and trace systems be for our residents, given our knowledge about issues such as barriers of language and trust?

Together, we looked at additional factors. Could we do more to support people with underlying health conditions? If people with diabetes had better management of their conditions, would that increase their resilience to Covid infection? What more could our GPs and primary care staff do to reach out to at-risk populations to try to ensure all were being supported? A lot of the work here was being led by Dr Muhammad "Wax" Naqvi, a GP from Forest Gate in the north of the borough, who like many others, worked tirelessly through the pandemic to try to address inequalities. He has long been determined to do so, but his motivation was enhanced by the loss of many patients and, in the first wave, a mentor and colleague and one of the many Black and Asian clinicians who lost their lives in the pandemic.

We tried to start addressing the issue of delayed access to care. We put up multi-language posters around the borough with the 12 most-spoken languages visible. Punjabi, Urdu, Hindi, French (for our large Francophone African population) and Lithuanian were among them. We launched a Covid helpline run by a local charity with multiple languages spoken and publicised it so people could have somewhere straightforward to dial into for Covid-related issues.

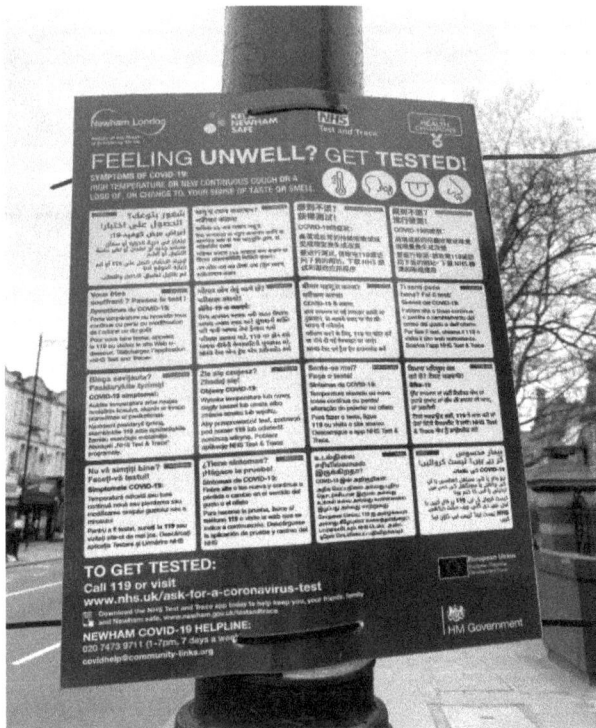

A "Feeling Unwell?" poster in 12 locally spoken languages.

Later on, when we established our local contact tracing service and had data on everyone who tested positive for Covid, we decided to do welfare calls. We would try to contact every single resident who tested positive for Covid in the first couple of days after their positive test. Again, as we developed this team, we ensured it had people who could speak our main community languages. Of the many things we would speak to people about, an important thing was making sure individuals knew how to access care if their symptoms got much worse.

As I said, we also had an eye on the long term. In areas such as Newham, organisations like the NHS and councils (and social care, although the council often isn't the direct employer) are major employers. They are always among the biggest in the borough. They are also disproportionately the employers of people from Black and Asian communities. Yet there was evidence of people employed by such agencies feeling powerless in their roles, as exemplified by the concerns around lack of access to PPE. This would be a problem we would have to address. The public sector can provide excellent employment, so we should be using our collective pounds not only to ensure good opportunities for our people, decent pay, and opportunities for progression in careers (not just to the most senior roles), but also to create environments where people feel respected, not judged due to the colour of their skin, and with the confidence to speak up.

We were just beginning this journey when Kevin Fenton's report was published in August 2020. It reiterated many of the concerns we had been working on and gave greater national prominence to addressing them. Critically, it shifted the lens. No more would the way we understood health inequalities in the UK exclude considering race and racism as a primary factor alongside poverty and class. It was now clear to us that, however the pandemic progressed, we would need to consciously consider this lived reality for so many of our residents. Most critically, we needed to talk to them.

As we reflected on these emerging issues early in the summer of 2020, Newham's mayor, Professor Fenton, and I discussed how we should address some of the factors that were concerning us. Through these conversations, the Covid Champions programme was developed; one of the most profound and impactful experiences of my pandemic.

Chapter 10
Champions

As we reflected on the first wave of Covid, its impact on our borough, the loss and devastation, and the extraordinary changes to people's lives, we knew we needed to change our approach to meet the challenges the pandemic would continue to throw at us.

One aspect we were clear on was the need to reach deeper into our communities, both to help people navigate the challenges and to understand the pressing concerns of our residents. We strongly suspected that – in the first wave – there were differences in understanding across our community about what was going on. As mentioned earlier, for example, how did people understand the government's slogan: "Stay Home, Protect the NHS, Save Lives"? Did some stay at home instead of attending hospital, as some of our doctors feared, when the NHS was exactly what they needed?

In many ways, lockdown was simple. There were few rules and little guidance to follow; essentially, we just had to stay at home. People in Newham, as in most places, overwhelmingly followed those simple rules, and the first wave (in terms of new infections) fizzled out quite quickly post-lockdown.

As lockdown eased, a slew of rules now came into force. Adam Wagner, the barrister who developed particular expertise in Coronavirus law, would – by February 2022 – identify 92 legislative updates to the UK coronavirus regulations. The rules were changing constantly, and there was rapidly changing advice on many aspects of life, from how to manage people's individual risks to where to find support.

Life was easing for many people, but at the same time, everything became increasingly complicated. Where can I go and with whom? When should I test? How do I get a test? How should I manage my underlying clinical vulnerability? What is NHS Test and Trace? Why should I trust them? If I need to isolate, can I get any help? What about my children?

Given all of the challenges of communication in Newham – multiple spoken languages, dozens of different communities, and minimal reliance on local media (many immigrants favour their home news channels and newspapers, for example) – how could we improve our communication with the community? We couldn't just keep putting up new posters on our streets every day in response to the latest changes, or rely on our council's Twitter feed or Facebook page, which reached tiny numbers of people. We needed to do something different.

When I was working in the aftermath of the Grenfell Tower fire disaster, I saw incredible levels of mistrust between members of the community and the state. This mistrust has subsequently been well documented by many of the bereaved and survivors, as well as the wider community. One exception that left a strong impression, however, was a programme called Community Champions. Here, people funded by the council, but employed by a local charity, worked to build relationships over time with the community. They supported committed residents to promote health in their neighbourhood, focusing on what they – the residents – were most passionate about. Equally importantly, the employed "champions coordinators" *listened*. They heard residents' issues and concerns and brought those community experiences back into the public health team and the wider council.

When I returned to my job in Camden and Islington in North London, I tried to establish similar programmes. It felt central to our purpose and values that public health shouldn't be a paternalistic endeavour (us professionals knowing what's best for people) but a collaboration of skills, passions, and energies working towards shared goals. When I arrived in Newham in April 2019, in my first role as director of public health, this was one of the first things I established. It was just starting out, working with a small number of residents on the important issue of poor air quality in Newham, when Covid hit. The programme was paused.

Rokhsana Fiaz, Newham's mayor, read voraciously on Covid throughout the pandemic, and would often send me links to SAGE (Scientific Advisory Group for Emergencies) and other academic papers that she thought I should read. She had come across a model of Community Connectors that had worked in the aftermath of the 2005 Hurricane Katrina disaster, acting as a trusted link between local government and community and helping people navigate the challenging environment of New Orleans post-Katrina. As we developed our plans for the ongoing pandemic, we discussed these approaches with Professor Kevin Fenton. Using our fledgling Champions model in Newham, and some learning about the New Orleans method as guides, we decided to embark on a new approach as we entered the next phase of the pandemic.

I brought in Anne Pordes-Bowers, an American expat with the perfect combination of skills for the job; a policy brain combined with a warm, empathetic approach and a strong commitment to the principles of community organisation and empowerment among her attributes. She wasn't from a public health background and knew no more than a typical layperson about Covid at that point. But that wasn't necessarily a problem. In fact, arguably, it was a virtue; she really could see the pandemic through the lay lens of our residents.

Anne took up the challenge. From the beginning, we were clear that this needed a very specific kind of approach. Where our pre-Covid fledgling health champions programme had worked with a relatively small number of people previously, aiming to collaborate with them in a deep and lasting way, we now needed to cast the net much wider. If that meant the relationship had to be a bit shallower, that was a necessary trade-off. We had a big population to reach and needed large numbers of people to deliver our model.

Anne invited a number of residents to form part of a group to design the programme together. What should it be called? How should it operate? What would residents want to get out of it?

Prior to Covid, almost all community meetings would have been held in person at town halls, libraries, or other community venues. We would have considered the idea of doing things online to be highly problematic, as – even if many people had the technology to do it (which they did not) – surely it would have excluded many others?

With many restrictions very much in place and Covid circulating, meeting virtually was the only option.

We got to work recruiting our residents to become involved. We put out messages through Twitter, took an ad in the local paper, and cascaded messages through our networks of community organisations and faith communities. Very quickly, people started to join.

Newham London
People at the Heart of Everything We Do

COVID-19
HEALTH
CHAMPIONS

Live or work in Newham?
Want to help stop the spread of coronavirus?
Become a COVID-19 Health Champion

How does it work?

1. You sign up to be a champion.

2. We give champions the latest information about COVID-19.

3. Champions share this information with anyone in their community, however they want.

4. Champions let us know what is and isn't working.

REGISTER TO BECOME A CHAMPION

🌐 www.newham.gov.uk/CovidHealthChampions
✉ CovidHealthChampions@newham.gov.uk
📞 020 3373 2777

OUR COVID-19 HEALTH CHAMPION MEETINGS

• **Thursday 18 June 6.30pm** with Jason Strelitz, Director of Public Health & Councillor Rohit Dasgupta
• **Wednesday 24 June 3pm** with Anne Bowers, Newham Public Health Team & Councillor Ann Easter
• **Saturday 27 June 3pm** with Jason Strelitz, Director of Public Health & Anne Bowers, Newham Public Health Team
More dates to follow

Find out more about being a COVID-19 Health Champion at:
www.newham.gov.uk/CovidHealthChampions

A Champion call-out.

The model hinged around two primary means of communication.

Twice (or sometimes three times) a week, we would run a Champions' Zoom call. Anne would host these, with her seemingly effortless charm, bringing laughter and smiles to this "serious" endeavour. We would use these calls to share updates and information with those present: what was happening to the case rate, what had changed in the response, and what might happen next.

Then, we would answer any questions. I, or colleagues from the public health team, would be there, and sometimes we would bring others – local GPs, a paediatrician, or others from the NHS, mental health specialists, or people from schools – to focus on different areas. It was an environment where anyone could ask anything. These meetings would build relationships and trust, give people deeper insight into the pandemic, and provide the opportunity to hear back from our residents about what they were feeling and the challenges they saw within the community.

Alongside this, we invited people to join a WhatsApp group. We would send out regular messages on different aspects of Covid safety and developed a model of infographics – very pictorial with few words – that could be easily cascaded through WhatsApp and Facebook. Over time, these would cover everything from basic Covid rules and safety messages to vaccine availability information and money advice. They were simple, and we would develop specific ones for particular events, such as Diwali, Eid, and Christmas (we even did one for Halloween), focusing on celebrating safely. They were kept simple so we could respond quickly to changes, such as new rules on testing or social distancing and new advice on shielding. Then, our Champions would share these through their networks. They were trusted messengers who could work with people we could never hope to reach.

Newham London
People at the Heart
of Everything We Do

KEEP NEWHAM SAFE

COVID-19
HEALTH CHAMPIONS

RULES ON MEETING WITH OTHERS

National Lockdown (from 5 November 2020)

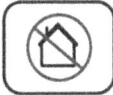

Meeting inside

- You cannot meet with people you don't live with inside your house or inside any public place.

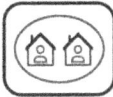

Some people can form a support bubble

- Households with only one adult (single person or single parent or carer families) can form a support bubble with another household.
- This means you can have close contact with that household as if they were members of your own household.
- Once you make a support bubble, you should not change who is in that bubble.

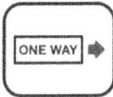

Being inside public buildings

ONE WAY

Follow all rules in COVID-19 safe venues including workplaces and schools. Any concerns can be raised with:
publichealthenquiries@newham.gov.uk

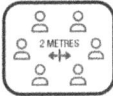

Being outside

2 METRES

- You can go outside with people you live with.
- You can go outside for exercise (eg walk, bike, jog).
- You can meet one person from outside your household/ support bubble on your own in an outdoor public place. You must stay 2 metres apart.

Keeping your distance helps keep others safe and **COVID-19** free

FOR QUESTIONS ABOUT COVID-19 OR HELP WITH ISOLATING:

020 7473 9711 (1-7pm, 7 days a week)

covidhelp@community-links.org

Example infographic.

Example infographic.

Our Covid Champions would do different things with the infographics. One person would send them to every mosque in the borough; another would print them out and stick them up on windows in their areas. Most people would promote them through their social and community networks.

The Champions programme took off. We built up a corps of 500 Champions, and although it was impossible to track how many we reached through the cascade, we know it was many thousands.

From the start, the Zoom calls combined an extraordinary lightness with deep seriousness of the endeavour. Emerging so soon after the devastating first wave, many of those who joined were recently bereaved, having lost people only recently in that first wave, including family members, friends, and community members. Many had lost several people. They wanted to share. In fact, for some, that was entirely the reason they wanted to participate. They did not want to be helpless, watching suffering in a continuing pandemic of an uncertain future, but determined to grasp some opportunity for agency… to make a difference in their community. As one participant said:

"It (the Champions programme) gives us the opportunity to contribute to our community, leaving us with a sense of self-worth and purpose during this difficult and isolating time."

At a time when I was highly stressed by the ongoing challenges of the pandemic, the evening Zoom calls with Champions were an oasis; a point of departure where we could just talk, reflect, be human together, each in our own way. Together, in these conversations, we tried to find a path through this extraordinary time in our lives, whatever our professional and personal circumstances.

We had an amazing diversity of ages and backgrounds, and a sense that we were creating something special. Quite quickly, news spread around the country about the Champions programme. Within a couple of months of launching, we had been inundated with requests from other areas eager to learn how to set up a scheme. Soon, there were dozens of these popping up all over the country.

With so much interest, I presented our work on a webinar to all the local authorities in the country, and Anne decided to establish a network of Champions coordinators (people doing her role) around the country to provide support to each other and share ideas. By October 2020, the government announced they were launching funding for a national scheme of Community Champions, with investment focused on different places across the country. Good ideas can often take years to spread; this one took months. It was incredibly exciting to see something we believed in so strongly be picked up so enthusiastically nationwide.

Over time, I got to know many of the Champions; locals such as Katie Blake, Lanre Odunlami, Joanne Dean, Iqbal Hussain, Oluwasegun Oyenigba and his son, Krystian Suliga-Oyenigba (a nine year old champion at the time), and many others in Newham who are amazing examples of people who just want to get involved in supporting their community. Sometimes, the state simply needs to give people a meaningful way to do so.

At the heart of this work was mutual respect and trust. From lots of feedback, I know that our residents felt valued and recognised because my colleagues and I prioritised the time to come and sit with them, answer their questions, and hear their concerns. But the feeling was entirely mutual. I think they knew that I was as grateful to them for taking the time to be part of our conversation, unpaid, out of their commitment to the community.

The gap between the state and citizens is widest when each believes the other's motives are different to their own. By building connections and relationships, it was clear that we were working towards the same goal; there was truly a shared endeavour. That's not to say there weren't disagreements, either between us or community members themselves. This kind of work isn't all warm and fluffy, but almost always, it was conducted in a spirit of mutual respect.

The true impact of the Champions was hard to measure. Our priority was to reach as many people as possible, so there were very low barriers to participation, no expectations of people, and no formal monitoring. We were trying to create an environment that was as enabling as possible. We did commission a report, *It Takes a Village: An External Review of the London Borough of Newham's COVID-19 Health Champions programme*, to try and capture some of the impact and much of it is best heard in the words of the Champions themselves.[21]

"I have access to a wide network of individuals from my community, and wanted to see if I could make a difference by knowledge sharing and making individuals whose first language isn't English aware of critical information related to the virus. I wanted to get involved and do something to help turn the tide on the pandemic and this was something I could do while working from home."

"Being part of the COVID Champions experience has empowered me in incredible ways. It's enabled me to become the 'go to' person for comms around COVID and I've been able to get my questions answered quickly and promptly without any judgement being made. It's also allowed me to share community concerns, particularly those affecting the ethnic minority communities and not feel 'embarrassed' by voicing such concerns."

"Being part of the Champions is inspirational. So many volunteers have been involved, it has been amazing to see how everyone worked as a team, valuing each other's strengths and abilities. I feel like my knowledge of the disabled community, language and cultural barriers has been valued. Because of my disabilities, I was made to feel like a problem in the community for years. The champion's programme hasn't made me feel like a problem, they have listened to me and asked me for advice on how to make the programme more accessible and inclusive."

"I know that the COVID-19 Champions Group has saved lives – even if it has saved one life (by encouraging someone to take the vaccine / by encouraging an elderly member of the community to self-isolate /

---

[21] See *It Takes a Village* - www.newham.gov.uk/downloads/file/4255/newham-covid-19-champions-evaluation-report-feb-2022

by giving out numbers where help can be obtained for accommodation) – lives have been saved. No matter what the social status, hand on my heart I can say 'help was there'."

Along the way, we learnt a lot. Doing this work on virtual platforms will clearly exclude some people; I will talk about the challenges of digital exclusion later. However, I suspect that it includes many more than it excludes. Popping onto a Zoom chat for an hour is a much smaller time investment than travelling to a community venue, sitting there for an evening, and then going home. For many people with caring responsibilities, health issues or disabilities, those who work late or face major barriers to community involvement, it made it far easier. It also made it easier for us, as it allowed community discussions to be put on multiple times per week with relative ease.

We learned how this work can build community itself. Those who got involved developed relationships with one another and others in their community. In the spring of 2021, after more than one year of only interacting over Zoom, some of us met for a picnic in the park. It was an emotional in-person connection of people from many different backgrounds; people who had shared an extraordinary journey together.

The strength of our community relationships and connections was, I think, one of the main reasons we were approached in late August 2020 and asked to pilot at short notice a new NHS Test and Trace app that was being developed. The app had been trialled once before, on the Isle of Wight earlier in the summer, with the trial indicating some potential but significant technological issues that needed resolving. Now, the developers believed those issues had been resolved and wanted to do some further pre-launch testing.

Wisely, they realised that the Isle of Wight was not fully representative of the country as a whole and looked for a more diverse, urban setting (it's hard to imagine somewhere in the UK much more different to the Isle of Wight than Newham). They had hoped to pilot in the North of England, but the region was enduring high rates of Covid at that point, and for those exact reasons, it was deemed unsuitable; they were too busy managing their situation.

So, they came to us. We weren't sure whether to participate either. I wasn't convinced about the efficacy of the tool, and we definitely had doubts about how our community would receive the app. We were also busy and tired from six long months of Covid response.

I was uncomfortable about going to our staff at zero notice and asking them to do a rapid, large piece of community engagement for something we weren't sure about. But we had resolved that we would do everything we could to protect the community, and while I knew it would be no panacea, I thought it might just be another helpful tool in our toolbox. Indeed, the chance to pilot the app and adapt it, based on the feedback from our residents, gave it the best chance of being something that would be useful locally. I also thought the resources we would get from NHS Test and Trace to publicise and promote the pilot would increase the likelihood that more of Newham's residents would download the app.

As I did multiple times through the pandemic, I turned to Rebecca Eligon, organiser of HelpNewham, as well as another "just gets stuff done" colleague, Ashlee Teakle. Implementing the same approaches, they brought people together and organised a community engagement sprint. We leaned heavily on the Champions, as well as other groups, as we needed thousands of people to download the app and then give us feedback. This is a challenge for a large local authority without significant media and communications channels.

The pilot was a qualified success. A lot of downloads were made, and discussions with the community and businesses gave useful feedback to the Test and Trace development team. The app was launched nationally a few weeks later with much fanfare and media buzz. All would then be relatively quiet with the app until the media-named "pingdemic" of summer 2021, when 600,000 people were alerted by their phone that they had been in close proximity to someone who had tested positive for Covid and needed to isolate for a week. How useful a tool it was remains unanswered.

Among other things, the pilot was a massive insight into the trust issues that existed in the wider community. Many people felt strongly that a tool such as the app, developed by the government, would be used for some nefarious purpose, such as their personal data being tracked and shared with authorities for reasons that had nothing to do with Covid.

Those issues of trust would become more and more significant as the pandemic wore on. The first six months of the Champions and the specific experience of the app pilot were valuable in themselves, but they would prove themselves to the greatest extent later in the year when we got to our most significant community challenge: rolling out the Covid vaccination programme. Even as the Champions programme rolled out nationally, this vaccination challenge was still some months away.

Chapter 11
Pubs Before Children

Nemesis, Philip Roth's novel set in 1940s New Jersey, captures the fear of death or disability that once stalked many communities, and specifically parents, before the widespread adoption of Jonas Salk's transformative polio vaccine.

"You washed the spit away but you didn't wash the polio away. You can't wash the polio away. You can't see it. It gets in the air and you open your mouth and you breathe it in and the next thing you got the polio."

Even in those times, when premature and childhood death was far more widely experienced as a fact of life, the fear was pervasive.

I've often reflected on how different our Covid experience would have been if the pathogen we were battling had been more harmful to children. The lockdowns and restrictions we experienced were, for many people anyway, crippling. But if children had been at greater risk – as with polio – those restrictions would have been significantly greater still.

However, as seemed clear from early on in the pandemic, children were spared the worst *direct* effects of the virus.

Despite that, if we accept Nelson Mandela's dictum that *"There can be no keener revelation of a society's soul than the way in which it treats its children"*, then UK society's response to Covid warrants some soul searching. When the dust finally settles on how the UK dealt with the enormous challenge of the pandemic, one of the areas (in fairness, there will be a few others) where we didn't get it right was with respect to our children and young people. As a nation, we did not sufficiently consider the needs of children when weighing up the impacts of pandemic management measures like school closures, nor did we adequately mitigate the effects on children of the measures we chose.

As with so many aspects of the Covid experience, in some ways, the impact on children and families was felt universally. Almost all families had the challenges of home schooling: the pale shadow of the vital, interactive social experience of normal school life.

As parents, we all had the challenges of keeping our children engaged or filling the many moments of boredom. We experienced worries about their social disconnection, concern over their wellbeing, and anxiety and guilty acceptance of the time they spent glued to screens. But, as with so many aspects of the pandemic, below the surface, people's experiences differed hugely.

Early in the pandemic, before lockdown, with a growing sense of what was to come, I went out to buy my son a new computer… he's going to need this, I thought to myself. Our home became replete with devices for everyone; we had effective broadband, and spaces for quiet study and individual online socialising. Alongside the privilege of a garden, these things didn't make lockdowns easy, but we did have some very valuable assets with which to navigate some of its challenges.

In Newham, however, 50% of children live below the poverty line. The main definition of poverty is a household with an income below 60% of the median income. For a family of two adults and two children, that is equivalent to less than £18,000 per year after housing costs. Managing on these levels of income is a significant strain. The evidence is clear that above a certain level of income, additional money is not associated with greater wellbeing. I may, in monetary terms, be far closer in income to someone on the minimum wage than I am to Elon Musk, or city bankers and lawyers, but my family is comfortably above the point of sufficiency and there is no evidence that increasing our income will improve our wellbeing.

Below the sufficiency level, however, life is hard. Daily struggles to increase income often mean working multiple jobs and facing tough choices about where to spend money. It means choosing between things that many of us take for granted – such as sufficient food, heating the home, and new children's shoes – and omitting certain basic needs for participating in modern life (like digital devices and money for decent broadband). In turn, the things that can take the strain from life, like breaks and holidays, treats, and help with childcare, are also foregone. Often, in places like East London, where property prices are extremely high and social housing is scarce, modern living is compounded by overcrowding. Many large families share small flats, and few have access to private gardens.

This was the backdrop for many in Newham when schools shut their doors to all, bar the children of key workers and others considered sufficiently vulnerable by children's social services.

Shutting schools raised a range of questions. What would be the impact on children who could not be well supported by their parents and carers at home, and for whom the nurture and support of teachers and staff at school was so important? What would be the impact on children who lacked decent computers and broadband to be able to participate in home schooling fully? What would be the impact on children who were reliant on their free school meals as part of their daily nutrition? What would be the impact on children when isolated from their peers for an extended period?

I could see some of this with my own eyes at home. While my children could have accessed school as the children of key workers, our eldest never wanted to, and our younger one (in primary school) grew less willing over time to be one of only a handful of children there. Yet my partner, a children's social worker, and I were far too busy with our work to be able to support them. It felt neglectful, but we told ourselves that as long as they were well and happy, we would just have to trust that whilst their academic development may have to take a hit – there would be plenty of chances to recover.

For many children and their families, however, the questions above played out in a far more challenging way.

Schools closed on March 23rd 2020, at the start of the first national lockdown. Despite plenty of discussion in the run-up to the closure, it wasn't clear that this would happen *until it did*. For us, as a local authority with a strong commitment to the wellbeing of our children and responsibility for child welfare and support to schools, we very suddenly had to grapple with these questions, too.

While vulnerable children were entitled to carry on attending school, there was considerable concern as to whether they would actually do so in sufficient numbers. Clearly, there was significant and understandable anxiety among parents, carers, and children themselves. With the absence of an evidence base, it was hard to confidently reassure anyone when many discourses circulating were anything but reassuring.

It wasn't clear, at first, how long school closures would last for, or how schools would manage remote learning. Neither, at this stage, had we gotten to grips with the technology of Zoom and Teams, which would soon become such a predominant feature of our lives. We were also deeply worried about inequitable digital access, as many of our families lacked digital devices or indeed broadband. Over time, there were some significant promises from central government, such as the delivery of 1.3 million laptops to children, but these were still being distributed towards the end of the third lockdown in April 2021; an incredibly slow translation into action. Local government simply didn't and doesn't have the resources in the way central government does to broach this digital divide.

By June 2020, as the levels of Covid had fallen to extremely low levels locally, I became convinced that schools should return in some way. My major concern was the separation and loneliness that children were experiencing. In the strange environment we were in, with many services being curtailed, it was hard to get quantifiable evidence on the impact on children, but from some of our Zoom conversations with young people, it was clear that many were feeling incredibly isolated.

At the same time, some challenges were hard to reconcile. For one, many school staff and their unions had deep concerns about the risks to their staff. This was understandable, particularly for those with clinical vulnerabilities who were still shielding, but what about staff returning home from work who lived with family members with clinical vulnerabilities? How could they manage the risk? Remember, these were still early days in understanding Covid transmission, and evidence was still emerging about ventilation and face coverings.

One issue touched me deeply. It emerged during a Zoom conversation with a group of school-age children as, along with colleagues, I tried to find out how things were going and what Newham's young people were concerned about. During this call, a number of young people shared their concerns about *returning to school*. Their anxiety was driven by the fact that they lived with older grandparents and other relatives who were shielding with underlying health conditions. These youngsters felt huge anxiety and fear that they risked catching Covid at school and bringing it home, carrying the risk into their family home.

As discussed earlier, this pattern of multi-generational living is commonplace in Newham but largely absent from much of the UK. These children were carrying immense worries that simply weren't shared by many others throughout the country. I couldn't help but feel the contrast to my own children. They were excited to return to school and be with their friends, with no real concerns about catching Covid because they knew that their young, healthy parents were at extremely low risk, and their grandparents were safely shielding in their own homes.

Like many issues in the pandemic, the issue of returning to school was one on which reasonable people could disagree, and neither answer was wholly palatable. We were dealing with a very challenging situation, and whatever choice was made, there would be some risks and costs – we needed to navigate them with thought and care and with a broad assessment of the relevant factors, listening to all the divergent voices.

I was asked to express my professional view as director of public health for the local area. This is what I wrote:

"As Director of Public Health for Newham, my absolute commitment is to support the health and wellbeing of our population, those who live and work in the borough. After the past few difficult and unprecedented months, with so much loss of life and the whole population impacted in deep ways, we are clearly entering a new phase of the pandemic.

The situation currently in Newham is undoubtedly far better than it was during the peak weeks of the pandemic. Our hospitals have few daily admissions for Covid-19, and the number of new positive confirmed cases is rising slowly.

However, we also know that the position is delicate. Newham was one of the last local authorities to have confirmed cases in London but was subsequently one of the most impacted by both numbers of cases and mortality. The risk factors which existed before the pandemic remain with us. We do not want to return to the situation of quickly rising numbers of cases which pose an immediate risk to the health of our population.

On the other hand, we know how important it is to children and families that aspects of normal childhood life resume: their education and connecting with friends is so important. Newham's schools make a major difference to the life chances of our children and we want them to continue with that vital role as soon as possible. My desire as Director of Public Health is for schools to return to supporting their children but in a safe way. I know that schools across the borough have already been doing a huge amount of work to support children of key workers and vulnerable children through the first phase of the pandemic, as well as preparing for this next phase.

Whilst Covid-19 is present in the UK, a sad reality for the foreseeable future, there are no guarantees of creating 100% risk-free environments; we all have to accept an element of risk when we go to the park, do shopping and increasingly now in this phase of lockdown as we reconnect with families and friends. Equally, the scientific advice is not definitive, we are learning all the time about a new virus and there are differences of opinion. We all, in both our professional and personal lives, have to navigate uncertainty.

What we all want for ourselves, our families, and friends is to be reassured that we are taking all the steps we can in a way that manages and reduces those risks as best we can.

In the context of schools, for me that means:

1. Not taking loosening steps until there is a low level of background risk in the community with the amount of Covid-19 low in our community.

The quality of data we have on the local epidemic in Newham is not as good as it should be and we have repeatedly asked Public Health England for more detail and timeliness in the data. However, based on the best evidence we have at the time of writing, there is a low level of infection risk in the community. This is not zero; the number of confirmed cases is going up but very slowly, and we anticipate this is an *underestimate of the real number. As lockdown eases, we expect these numbers will rise, albeit we hope slowly. Self-isolating when people have symptoms and following guidelines on social distancing and hygiene will be our best tools to limit spread further.*

2. That the local authority, including public health and the education team and NHS colleagues, are working closely with schools to support them in being Covid-19 ready and that schools themselves feel sufficiently equipped to manage risks for their staff, children and wider schools community.

We are working closely with schools around guidance and risk assessments. We will provide all advice as necessary to support them both individually and through webinars, and the completed toolkit, in taking these steps and are working with colleagues on a clinical advisory panel. This work is going on but there is clearly more to do, and we will continue to work with schools on an ongoing basis. Schools need to feel that their risk assessments are robust and be in a position to adapt them as they learn from the new challenges of providing school in this context.

3. That there is a robust track and trace system in place so we can be confident where local cases arise that they do not lead to outbreaks.

NHS Test and Trace is in an early stage of development, only launched last Thursday and will take some time to be fully embedded. This poses a significant challenge for us in Newham, as it does elsewhere, not just to schools but the wider context of community risk. Given this is not fully in place, and may not be for some time, and we cannot be assured of when we will feel confident in the national system, we ask schools to proactively contact us to discuss situations of concern around symptomatic children or staff or any confirmed cases in their schools so we can work alongside you to manage risk.

There remains uncertainty and we ask schools to continue to work closely with us around developing and learning how to operate in as safe a way as possible.

4. Respecting parental choice.

The range of risk factors that exist for different families in the borough, means that all will need to work out, for now, how to navigate risk and uncertainty for them. We need to ensure that families are not judged for their decisions and that children are well supported educationally, whether or not they physically attend school.

5. Readiness to change course.

Given the uncertainty over the state of the epidemic and the capability for it to change quickly, we need to be ready to change position not just in response to any localised outbreak but also a worsening situation in terms of the local epidemic.

Given this, while we recognise that schools nationally have been asked to take certain steps, I am of the view that schools should open to more children in a tentative and careful way, mindful of the ongoing work needed, and to work closely with Newham public health team on any emerging concerns, but also with a view that if we have evidence of the situation deteriorating locally to be ready to change course even if the national position is different."

So, despite the concerns of some school staff and children, I was sure that schools should start to return, even if it meant that some people's risks would have to be managed in different ways. The majority needed a return. My thinking on this was threefold.

Firstly, at this point, the risk had clearly diminished hugely. The borough had suffered terribly through the first wave, but the case rate was now very low, and in particular, clinical risks to children we now knew were low. It appeared that children – particularly at young ages – didn't even become infected, let alone become seriously unwell.

Secondly, at this point, there was no great confidence in the timeline for effective vaccination. We were still in the early days of the pandemic, so insisting that we wait for an effective vaccine to be rolled out across the population meant that we could be waiting indefinitely.

Thirdly, I was convinced, from all the evidence and the expert briefings I was receiving, that there would be new waves later in the year. If we couldn't return to school at this low level of case rate and transmission, when could we? We had to start somewhere, otherwise our children could be out of school for a very long time with hugely significant consequences.

For many children, though, schools never reopened for the 2020-2021 academic year. When pubs reopened on July 4th, on what some newspapers referred to as "Freedom Day", allowing us adults to get together with our mates once more to enjoy a sociable beer, it was a wonderful relief. But it was clear to many people that, as a society, we had got something wrong; surely we weren't really opening pubs before schools? A month later, pub openings were followed by the launch of "Eat Out to Help Out", a government discount scheme to subsidise restaurant meals.

One of the deep frustrations at this point was the absence of an evolving plan by central government. Despite schools being closed for a couple of months, there seemed to be no clarity of vision, energy, or creative thinking centrally. There were clear differences between schools in their approaches, but all of them were operating within a tightly constrained national policy environment that didn't seem focused on finding ways of getting children back to school to some degree. This was summer 2020; we could do things outside.

We could split classes to reduce risk and maintain some social distancing. We could continue to protect those with the highest risk. But the focus on getting children back to school just didn't seem to be there in national policy.

To borrow the expression, to have one unplanned-for school closure could be considered unlucky; to have a second seemed inexcusable. But that was exactly what happened in January 2021 as we were trying to manage that devastating wave of Covid. On the positive side, six months on, schools were much more adept at supporting remote learning, and most were comfortable with new technologies. However, the same systemic challenges for disadvantaged children were still equally present. Plus, this was now the second lockdown, and in winter, which was to be so much harder in many ways.

I don't subscribe to the view that this second closure shouldn't have happened. I understood the need for school closures at this point. In January 2021, we were in the midst of a horrific second wave, vaccinations had only just begun, and by controlling some transmission, we were saving lives. But we also knew a lot more. In particular, we knew how little transmission occurred outside and how safe it remained for children. We could easily have allowed children to come together for sport and physical activity, to come together to connect socially and have contact with professional adults outside their families. It felt as if policymakers thought that allowing children to play football at this point would set a bad example for the rest of society, sending out the message that coming together was okay. It felt like one particular view of behavioural insights was once again having an undue impact.

But that's not how I saw it or how it was in other countries that were equally trying to manage transmission. Other countries took a broader view of risks, weighing up the specific risks of Covid infection and transmission against those of our children's physical and mental health and development, and in doing so chose to curtail children's lives less; we might have taken more notice of their views.[22] International research on the consequences of school closures on children during the pandemic has shown the profound impact they have had on both learning, and physical and mental health.[23]

I think one of my personal biggest regrets of the pandemic was not doing enough to think more creatively about how to mitigate risks. There is widespread concern that the pandemic had an impact on children and young people's educational attainment, alongside aspects of their development, mental health, and wellbeing. These impacts are always distributed unevenly, with the least advantaged bearing the greatest cost. I have no doubt we could have done more to mitigate these risks, even while we took necessary steps like school closures. If an event similar to Covid happens again, we must do things differently. We must plan appropriately, mitigate harms wherever possible, and maintain a firm focus on those most likely to be adversely impacted.

---

[22] See, for example, Lindblad, S., Wärvik, G.-Band and others (2021). School lockdown? Comparative analyses of responses to the COVID-19 pandemic in European countries. *European Educational Research Journal*, *20*(5), 564-583.

[23] Mazrekaj, Deni, and De Witte, Kristof. The impact of school closures on learning and mental health of children: Lessons from the COVID-19 pandemic. *Perspectives on Psychological Science* 19.4 (2024): 686-693.

Chapter 12
Barriers to Isolation

When we finally got access to the data about who was testing positive for Covid, it was a game-changer. We had argued for a long time that we needed it, and once the data started to arrive, that data came in a deluge. We went from "flying blind" to having, we thought, a pretty complete picture of local infections.

Eventually, we had information on all the confirmed cases reported to NHS Test and Trace and any close contacts that those individuals had identified. We quickly got to work considering what we could do to complement the work of NHS Test and Trace meaningfully.

NHS Test and Trace, as discussed earlier, was the often-mocked (possibly because, from day 1, it was hubristically referred to as "world class") national system for contact tracing, which was established at huge expense. In truth, I was positively surprised at how successful it seemed to be at reaching Newham's population. My pessimistic assumption had been that the language barriers and cultural distance between a national call centre and Newham's population would be too great to make it remotely effective. However, the data we received suggested it successfully connected with four out of every five cases they tried to reach.

We didn't want to simply duplicate the work of NHS Test and Trace; we needed to add value to what they were already doing. There were three main concerns which guided our thinking.

The first was, obviously, the one in five of our population that Test and Trace was not reaching. Could we make an additional effort once they had tried to reach people – to follow up and use local data, community languages, contacts, and perhaps home visits – to try to ensure we were reaching everyone?

The second was a deeper concern. While the data we received suggested that NHS Test and Trace successfully got through to cases, further information suggested that those conversations generated only a tiny number of contacts. Contact tracing is an important tool in the management of infectious diseases, so understanding who the likely contacts of a positive case are, and then advising them in a way that aims to limit further spread, is key. If NHS Test and Trace wasn't identifying many contacts, then it raised questions about their approach, the main one being whether the calls themselves were terribly effective… a possible example of "hitting the target but missing the point". Perhaps they were getting through to people, but the communication or trust issues I suspected a national call centre would face were limiting the effectiveness of the conversations.

I had experienced many of these kinds of conversations during my public health training, following up on people who had tested positive for various infections such as E. coli or hepatitis B, and I followed a clear protocol depending on the infection and the situation. In all my time doing these phone calls, I can't remember ever discussing how likely it was that people would actually follow the advice that I, or my colleagues, had given them. It felt like an unspoken assumption within the field that advice and guidance would be heeded; we never discussed what barriers people may face in taking forward recommended actions.

Back with Test and Trace, how much were the callers building a rapport with those they were speaking to? Were they explaining *why* this mattered and showing empathy for their situation to build that trust? I just didn't know. It was impossible to get beneath the skin of the ultimately superficial performance data we were receiving; it just told us how many people they were getting through to and how many contacts they were generating. I raised this issue several times in meetings with regional and national colleagues, and people would nod in agreement, but we could never get meaningful evaluation data.

The third concern went deeper still. Contact tracing is part of public health orthodoxy in the management of communicable diseases. It is clearly an effective strategy in many situations, invaluable, for example, in managing risk around something like HIV, both in trying to control spread but also alerting people to their own potential risk (a subset of contact tracing referred to as "partner notification"). But how effective was it for Covid? Among my concerns was the sheer volume of cases that were 'out there' about which we had no idea. At this stage, in late summer 2020, there were no widely available lateral flow tests and no asymptomatic testing. Therefore, those showing up in our Test and Trace data were the tip of our Covid iceberg. Moreover, it was clear that a large percentage of Covid transmission was from people showing no symptoms, passing on infections before they were ever tested (if they ever were).

The implication was that we were contact tracing on a tiny subset of cases, so even if it was highly effective with those people, we knew it was highly limited in controlling the spread of the infection among the wider population. That didn't necessarily make it totally redundant; it was just a much blunter tool in our toolbox than for other situations. You are essentially trying to play whack-a-mole with a small number of cases and giving focused attention to them.

Once we started to call people, I wondered whether other aspects of those conversations were equally or more important than contact tracing.

We rapidly developed our local contact tracing service under the leadership of experienced environmental health officers who deeply understood the challenges of having these kinds of sensitive conversations with residents. Many of the EHOs had followed up in Newham's communities when people were identified with certain infections over the previous years. They worked with my colleague Lizzie Owen, who had developed conversation scripts months earlier when we had started HelpNewham (our self-isolation support service).

When we developed HelpNewham, we knew it was important to identify those who genuinely didn't have any other support they could rely on. This was because, with our limited resources, there was no way we could support everyone. At the same time, we were equally committed to ensuring that people who did need support wouldn't be embarrassed or too proud to say so. We knew that many would be, so it was vital to develop rapport and trust with these residents, even though we were essentially cold-calling them. Lizzie brought her skills and sensitivities to the task of developing our contact tracing scripts.

As it turned out, our thinking crystallised around an approach I spotted on Twitter (I used Twitter a lot during the pandemic!). Firstly, I found it a constant source of wisdom and insight. The regular threads of expertise from people like Professors Devi Sridar and Christina Pagel from the University of Edinburgh and UCL, respectively, kept me informed and challenged, up-to-date with the latest emerging evidence base, and in touch with critical thinking on the country's strategic approach to the pandemic.

I also used Twitter as one way to cascade messages into the community. While it reached small numbers in absolute terms, it felt like lots of people engaged in community leadership were active in that virtual space. Their engagement felt worthwhile (although likely of limited effectiveness, given the small number of people I would reach locally). As mentioned earlier, I also used it for raising my concerns when I was feeling alarmed by developments.

But I think I used it most frequently to share positive stories about what we were doing. I thought it important to celebrate our different projects and the work of our colleagues across the council, NHS, and community organisations. Through my tweets, I looked to keep people informed, sharing positive stories in largely grim times.

A relatively small number of fellow directors of public health used Twitter regularly in a similar way. It was one of them, Lisa McNally, the DPH in Sandwell in the West Midlands, who tweeted when she launched Covid Welfare Checks, a programme that augmented their local contact tracing with phone calls to ensure people were in okay health, and ascertain whether they needed additional support.

This approach resonated strongly with me. As discussed earlier, one of my major concerns in the aftermath of the first wave had been that people had not been quick enough to access medical help when their Covid symptoms were becoming significantly worse. As I touched on earlier, we had created a highly unusual mechanism for dealing with Covid, bypassing the UK's long-established norms of healthcare behaviour. Typically, when we are unwell (unless it seems like an emergency), we go to our GP. They will diagnose, advise, and potentially treat, and we will definitely leave with guidance on what to do if our condition deteriorates. With Covid, we just went to get tested if we had symptoms, and we essentially received a laboratory report telling us if we were either positive or negative, plus some guidance. People didn't have any actual conversations with health professionals about their situation. What would they do if they lacked the knowledge or confidence of what to do if they became increasingly unwell?

So, alongside the contact tracing we would carry out to augment Test and Trace, we decided (based on Sandwell's example) to do welfare checks as well, as soon as we knew of people's diagnoses. Alongside our voluntary sector-run helpline, this was our own Covid Support Service. We were conscious that residents might find this a duplication (in truth, people seemed to get called incessantly by NHS Test and Trace), but most seemed to realise our calls were different, and we received very few complaints. Instead of being focused on getting information out of people and telling them what to do, these calls were about giving them advice and seeing if they had support needs.

Our call handlers were local to the area, having been redeployed from other council services like our libraries and council tax advisors, and knew what support was available in the local community. They also spoke many of Newham's different languages and were trained to provide very basic health advice, so people knew what to do if their symptoms deteriorated.

Through all this, we were able to understand the needs of the community. Some people were feeling particularly isolated, so we could connect them with Chat Newham, the volunteer-led befriending service we had created in the early days of the pandemic. Other people were struggling to get food as they didn't have people to bring them shopping, and it was hard at this stage of the pandemic to get deliveries. As such, we organised food supplies through the distribution hub we had developed.

The biggest concern, however, was finance. We had identified this as a risk long before the government introduced the Test and Trace Support payment, a temporary addition to the country's social security system to help people in work to self-isolate. The burden of isolating or caring for others was significant in an area with low financial resilience and many people living week-to-week, covering rent, bills, and basic needs (alongside zero-hours contract work or other less-protected employment). We introduced hardship grants, administered by a local charity, to try to ensure that people could afford to take public health action (isolating for the benefit of others) without facing a significant financial penalty.

This was another time when I was acutely conscious of my privileges during the pandemic. Not only was I able to work from home, as most affluent workers could, but I had an employer who would look after me if I became unwell and couldn't work. Many employees in Newham may have been in the same choppy sea, but our boats couldn't have been more different in terms of employment and income. While I was essentially on a cruise ship, totally unaffected financially should I or any of my loved ones come down with Covid, many residents in Newham – such as those on a minimum wage or with fewer permanent employment rights – were essentially in a rubber dinghy, at the whim of the storm.

Our Covid Support Service spoke to tens of thousands of residents throughout the pandemic. Every week, they would send me short case studies so I could understand the issues they were grappling with and, more importantly, the challenges our residents were facing. Here are some examples:

"I spoke to a gentleman on Tuesday who is a part of a family of eight and has just started a new job. As he is on probation, he is not entitled to sick pay. He made an application for a £500 support payment [national payment] *but was informed he wasn't entitled to it. I gave him some other options to get in touch with the Renewal Programme (a local charity we were working with) for a micro-grant and also with Our Newham Money (the council's welfare advice service), who might be able to offer other financial advice. He was pleased as he couldn't afford not to have income coming in for the next couple of weeks."*

"I spoke to this guy and feel really bad for him. He was doing a little bit of painting work here and there, but can't do anything cause he is now isolating. (I think he was barely making anything before.) He doesn't claim any benefits because he said he doesn't know how to go about doing things like that. He has been unable to pay his rent, so he

has been made to sleep in the lean-to of the building he was painting. He doesn't have a proper bed and he said it's really cold in that space and he doesn't think he is going to make it (which was obviously quite distressing to hear). He also hardly has any food."

"I spoke with a lady who told me she comes from Uzbekistan. She has three children, an 8 and 4-year-old and a 5-month-old. Her husband was told that he was not eligible for the £500 support payment. Her husband lost money when he had to isolate, as he was in training for a new job. They don't receive housing benefit either, and they've been told they don't qualify for Universal Credit even though she has been here since 2011 and her husband since 2006. They can't pay their rent. The landlord has given them 45 days to pay. They are really struggling to pay for food and pay the bills. She wasn't asking for help but I really felt she needed it, and so I helped her make an application to the Newham Food Alliance (the council food hub we had established) and to the Renewal Programme."

The extent of the isolation challenges that our residents felt made us sure this would stop many from testing in the first place. If testing, and the risk of a positive test, led to a choice between doing what you knew was the right thing to do (to not risk spreading Covid) or meeting the basic needs of paying rent and putting food on the table, wouldn't you just avoid testing in the first place? All of us try to avoid that level of dissonance and internal moral conflict.

Emerging insights about people's "barriers to isolation" made us want to understand these challenges further. We wanted to explore matters with greater rigour and share our findings more widely. In the middle of the time-pressured, reactive work of pandemic management, doing research can seem hard, even indulgent, when there are immediate challenges. Nonetheless, it is vital. How much better off are we for the quality research done on vaccines and treatments for Covid which started early? Because of this research, we didn't get lost down the garden path of "promising" intuitively sensible treatments; instead, researchers discovered those that were more effective and those that were not.

Yet, in the sphere of social rather than biomedical interventions, action-oriented research is much more limited. Indeed, for all the resources that get spent in local government, far too little is invested in meaningful applied research to ensure that we sufficiently understand the challenges we are grappling with. Only by comprehending these challenges can we deploy our limited resources in the most effective ways to address them.

Having said all this, there was nothing overly complex about the research we carried out at the time. We simply started asking people who called our Covid helpline. This research confirmed what we had picked up through our daily contact with thousands of residents. The initial barrier was all about testing…

"And I was telling him… have you got any symptoms of Covid? And they say to me, Oh yeah, I think I got it. And I said, why are you not calling NHS for any testing. And he said, no, I don't want to, because in case I'm positive and have to self-isolate. And, also, I couldn't do that because I have no recourse to any public funds and I don't get any benefits. So, if I lose my job I have, how can I survive? How can my family survive?"

Whilst mental health, isolation, and how to get hold of food were all prominent worries, the number one concern for people, when it came to following government advice ("test, trace and isolate"), was that they would lose their job if they were forced to take time out of work.

I thought I had some understanding of the lack of financial resilience that people had, through the nature of poverty and our low pay end of the labour market, plus the hand-to-mouth existence that many in our community faced. Still, it came as a shock to hear how many people perceived themselves to be in such fragile and unsupported employment. The contrast between my personal experience and that of many of our residents could not have appeared any sharper. To ask them to make decisions that policymakers essentially viewed as minor inconveniences or, at worst, a small pain left me cold. And while we could talk with policymakers about small amounts of financial support, mental health, and access to food, labour rights simply weren't part of any discussion.

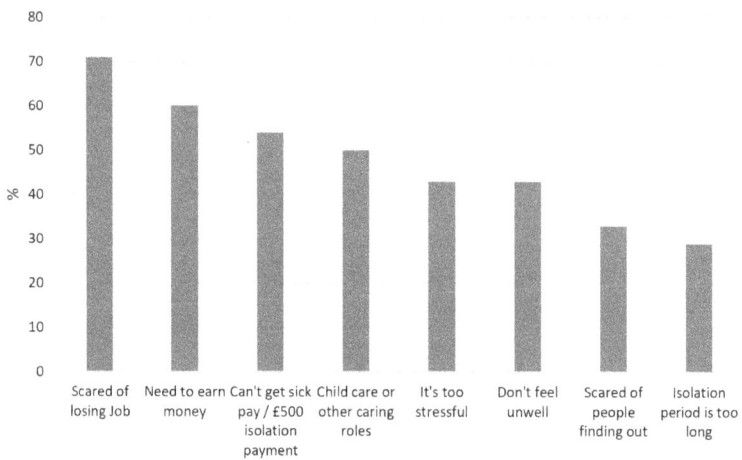

What do you think gets in the way of people being able to isolate (stay at home) if they have COVID-19 or are a contact of someone with COVID-19 (n=129). Source: Newham / University of East London Research (Feb 2021)[24]

Since the first wave, one of the other areas where we considered Newham's population particularly exposed was in housing. As discussed earlier, Newham has especially high levels of overcrowding, making it incredibly difficult for a Covid-positive household member to isolate from others.

---

[24] Newham Council/University of East London (2021) What helps, what gets in the way of being able to self-isolate?

Furthermore, one particular feature of inner urban areas with large multi-ethnic populations, as described in the previous chapter on children, is that they are also far more likely to be multi-generational: older parents tend to live with their adult children and families.

Young adults, due to the socio-economic context, are more likely to be in jobs where they are out and about in the community and more likely to be exposed to infection. Older adults, meanwhile, are more likely to have underlying health conditions, exposing them to greater risk if they catch an infection. All in all, this setup represented an elevated cocktail of risk.

But this was an issue that did not enter into national policy thinking. Partly because it was a difficult problem to solve, but probably more so because it simply didn't impact most of the British population. Nationally, this mix of overcrowded and multi-generational housing was limited to a relatively small number of areas, but for Newham, it was a significant issue.

So, from our initial plans following the first wave, we talked about how we could mitigate risk. Naturally, we knew that we would struggle to overcome the challenge of overcrowded housing over the course of a generation, let alone in the months of a pandemic.

Our ideas started to develop significantly with the introduction of rapid asymptomatic testing at the beginning of 2021. Prior to this, the only tests available were laboratory PCR tests. With PCR, by the time someone experienced symptoms, then tested, and then received the results back from NHS Test and Trace, it was likely that any window for intervention had gone. Chances were, positive residents would have spread Covid around households already. However, with rapid asymptomatic testing, perhaps we could identify people much earlier and intervene before they had passed on the infection.

When rapid testing began, my colleague, Claire Greszczuk, set up an amazing network of rapid testing sites throughout the borough. Utilising a number of libraries and community centres, she ensured that every person in Newham could walk to a test site and receive the support needed to do a rapid test. As was consistent with our ethos, the sites were supportive, building connections with the residents who used them. We tried to ensure that people knew the different kinds of support they and their families could receive if they tested positive.

When the testing programme started, we immediately tried to target those in multi-generational housing. We used council data to identify homes and tried to promote messaging so people would understand how rapid testing could help them mitigate risks. It was a hard message to communicate; this technology was new, and we understood that it takes time for people to hear about and digest the potential benefits.

With this ability to test proactively and receive results almost immediately, we returned to an idea we had considered at the first wave's end. Could we support people in multi-generational homes to isolate themselves in hotels while they were infectious?

There was a clear rationale for this, but it simply wouldn't work without the rapid tests; the intervention would be too late. Now, though, we could give it a proper test.

Working with our colleagues from the local authority housing team, we found a number of hotels that we could use and set about trying to promote the offer. Clearly, it wasn't as simple as just offering a hotel room. If that person was to be isolating, we would need to ensure that they had access to food, prescriptions, and – if necessary – mental and physical health support. Moreover, if they were a caregiver to elderly parents, we would need to make sure there was someone able to continue doing that; otherwise, people would not take up the offer in the first place.

Although it was a plan fraught with complexity, we managed to get the Newham hotel isolation support up and running. It intrigued people and got quite a lot of publicity, even a write-up in the *New York Times*.[25] But it was very slow to be utilised. Mostly, I think it was just too far outside the cultural norms of the people. When faced with a health challenge, their instincts weren't to stay in a hotel but to be at home. Furthermore, people are particularly reluctant to leave elderly relatives.

Without it being a national policy (just something we tried to promote locally), it was hard to get sufficient numbers of people to know about the scheme and think of it as a mainstream approach. Perhaps, also, when we finally got it off the ground, the vaccine programme had started and it was just too late to make a real difference. We maintained the offer for many months, and it would be used increasingly over time, but never in large numbers. Nevertheless, we still felt good about it. Our commitment had been to try to use every tool we could think of to protect our community, combating every risk we could. Housing was clearly one of these risks, and we had tried to find something to mitigate its effects.

Throughout the pandemic, this "inequality in isolation" was profound. Isolation was a policy that appeared to be a straightforward ask for many in our population, including myself and my family, yet it was fraught with complexity for many others. Whether it was household overcrowding, multi-generational living, low wages, insecure employment, or a

---

[25] Pandemic Needs Its Smokey Bear, *New York Times*, 8 March 2021

lack of familial support, it was clear that a range of factors shaped people's choices in profound ways.

Chapter 13

Clapping for the NHS:
The Rise and Fall of Solidarity
in The Pandemic

One particularly memorable ritual of the early days of the pandemic was the weekly clap for the National Health Service (and latterly care workers). Across the country, at 8pm on a Thursday, we rose from our dinner tables or left whatever we were watching on TV, piled out of our homes (some with pots and pans to bang) and lined the streets to clap for our "NHS heroes" (it was very much the NHS at first). My family participated religiously.

As well as thanking those workers, it was about acknowledging what everyone was going through, a weekly ritual that marked the unprecedented times we were in and, like most rituals – religious or otherwise – something that was particularly meaningful because it was communal. We did it together.

I remember, in the early days of "the clap", wondering when it would ever end. With the pandemic in full throttle, increasingly despairing evening news, no vaccine, and no end in sight, I genuinely thought we might be doing this new ritual for many years to come. When would it be ok to stop?

But it did stop, and quite abruptly. This "clap" actually only happened for ten weeks, from the first Thursday after lockdown began until the end of May.

Although I'd been a fan, I was mostly ok with it ending for two reasons. Firstly, at least in London, we were – by that tenth week – in a calmer phase of the pandemic. The first peak's attack speed was matched by its decline post-lockdown. The emergency Nightingale Hospital in Newham had been mothballed earlier in the month, having taken few patients, and while NHS staff remained exhausted and significantly stretched, we felt we were past the worst. Our greatest fears subsided; better days were ahead.

Secondly, a bit of a professional backlash had started to occur towards "the clap". Some argued that "we don't need a clap; what we need is decent pay which recognises our contribution." A reasonable refrain, particularly from lower-paid public sector workers who had seen many years of real-term stagnation in their wages. For others, the backlash was about being more inclusive. Many, including NHS staff, objected to being singled out. This was most blatant for care workers, who faced similar challenges and risks (if not greater, as subsequent data showed) and who are forever marginalised in political and public discourse compared to their NHS counterparts. However, many also highlighted the vital role that other staff were playing, keeping the country going but facing risks and being unable to work from home, such as bus and train drivers and supermarket workers, to name just a few.

A further critique came from those who simply said we are not heroes; we are just doing our job, and it's been awful. In discussions with some hospital staff, I was introduced to "moral injury", a concept that gained traction for NHS and care workers during the pandemic. While this meant different things to different people, what I understood was that the enormity of the challenges of Covid – the lack of knowledge to treat early patients, a shortage of equipment, and the basic insufficiency of their actions – put them into psychological conflict with their sense of self as clinicians, particularly in the early days of the pandemic. Their identity was to help people, but they simply couldn't do so in the way that felt right.

The summer drifted on well for those of us in London. I was acutely conscious of colleagues in the Midlands and North, initially Leicester and then much of the North West, where the first wave had peaked later. By the time some aspects of lockdown started to ease, they hadn't seen a sufficient fall in numbers and their rates quickly picked up again. While I got some respite, including a lovely week in Wales with my family, they were managing ongoing larger numbers of cases (in time, these numbers would seem trivial compared to later surges in the pandemic).

Infections in London had remained low through July and August but clearly picked up at the beginning of September 2020 as both schools returned and people slowly began to return to their offices. Through the early autumn, cases rose steadily, though not at the alarming pace of the previous March. There remained a huge number of restrictions on social contact in our lives.

As the rates of Covid infection increased again in the autumn, in the wake of what had felt to most people like a welcome relaxation of restrictions, including "Eat Out to Help Out" and the start of the new school year, I started to miss "the clap" or, at least, the solidarity it represented. In a tweet towards the end of September, I channelled Joni Mitchell, *"Don't it always seem to go, that you don't know what you got 'til it's gone"* and wrote:

"Short thread on solidarity - been thinking about the weekly clap and as much as it was an expression of thanks to NHS, care workers and others, it was also about communal solidarity — feeling connected with our families and neighbours that we were navigating this challenge together.

Feels like the discourse has become too focussed on non-compliance but measures from isolation to face coverings are for many people about protecting others as much as if not more than self & therefore must be rooted in positive sense of community not just coercion.

Many NHS workers were touched by the clap but others didn't want to be on a pedestal, but what about we clap for everyone — young people missing out on rites of passage, people out of work or struggling on reduced pay, more clinically vulnerable worried about the next phase?

Many of us are feeling a dip in energy and confidence as we try to steel ourselves to do this again and this time through winter – can't help feeling it would be easier if we remembered we are all in this, not all in the same way as each other, but not no one is unaffected – why don't we clap for everyone?"

I can't say this was my most successful tweet of the pandemic, but it resonates strongly with me to this day. As the tweet implies, it wasn't the clap, per se; it was the shift from a collective sense of purpose (which characterised the early days of the pandemic) to a more individualistic narrative that had increasingly taken root. Features of solidarity in the early days were not just the clap, but the mutual aid groups trying to meet people's needs on their streets and in their neighbourhoods, the tens of thousands of people volunteering for the NHS, and the ubiquitous rainbows children drew and displayed in their windows.

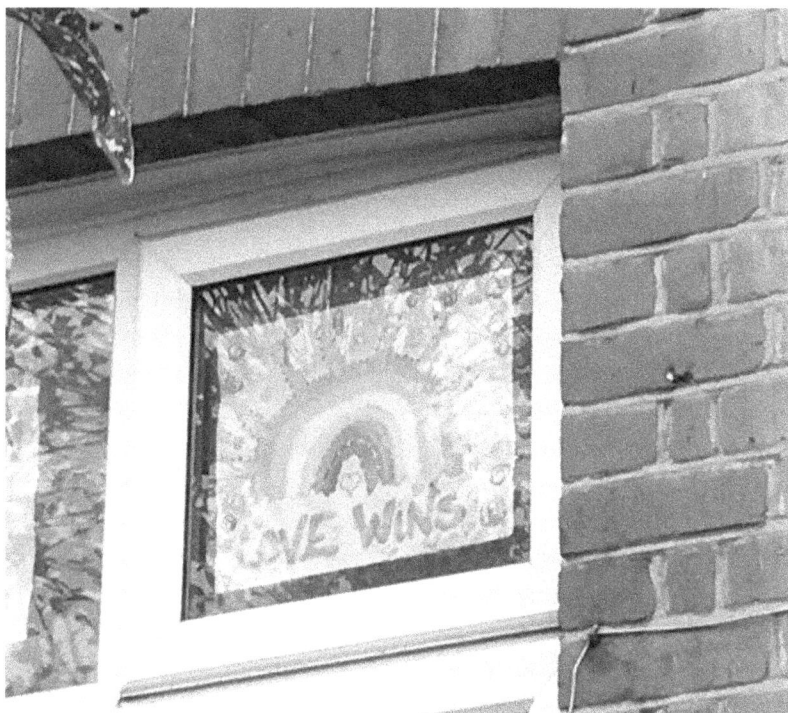

Solidarity rainbow posters were common in home windows for many months.

As the tweet articulated, I felt that the narrative had shifted to focus on individual behaviour. However, those behaviours we were asking people to comply with were predominantly to protect others rather than themselves. Yes, there were things we could do to protect the people we knew and loved, but much of the purpose of both recommended measures and compulsory restrictions was to restrict the circulation of the virus generally; to protect strangers as much as ourselves and loved ones. If we didn't have a sense of collective purpose, how would we maintain the willingness to make individual sacrifices for the common good?

What might have precipitated this shift away from collective purpose?

In some sense, this was just normal. When I worked as part of the Grenfell Tower Fire Disaster recovery, I became familiar with the Red Cross's post-disaster trajectory, which is a representation of a prototypical emotional response to a disaster. It depicts fear and anticipation followed by a collective desire to act (with a "honeymoon" peak in social cohesion), followed by an extended period of fatigue and disillusionment, then a slow return to the pre-disaster baseline, punctuated by difficult moments.

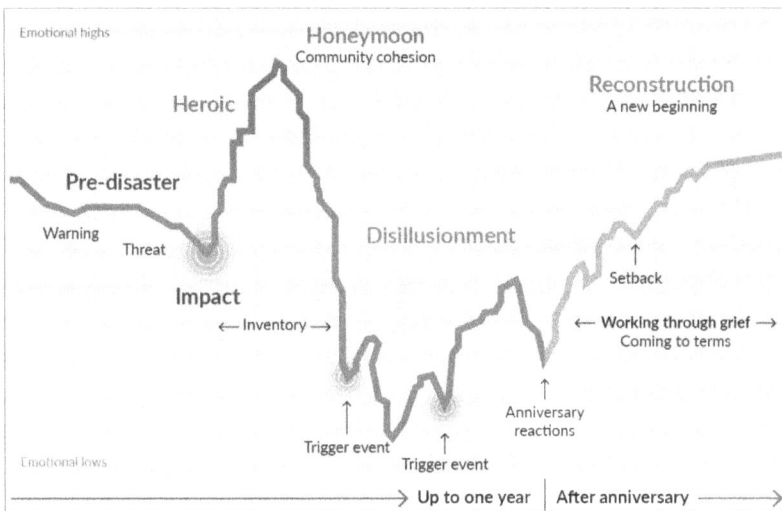

The path to recovery following a traumatic event. From "Covid-19 recovery and resilience: what can health and care learn from other disasters?" courtesy of The King's Fund (used with permission).[26]

26   https://features.kingsfund.org.uk/2021/02/covid-19-recovery-resilience-health-care/ derived from Myers D, Zunin L (2000). 'Psychological reactions to disaster' in DeWolfe DJ (ed). *Training manual for mental health and human service workers in major disasters,* 2nd ed. Washington DC: Federal Emergency Management Agency and Substance Abuse and Mental Health Services Administration.

The period from March 2020, the first days of the pandemic, through the first couple of months was absolutely typical of the heroic/honeymoon phases of normal disaster responses. We all came together with a sense of cohesion and common purpose. Our response to the initial shock was to strive for control and agency; we wanted to make a difference. In many disaster contexts, this is when donations pile up, money is raised, and people volunteer if they can. We saw it again, post-pandemic, when Russia invaded Ukraine. There was a surge of concern, with fundraisers, vigils, and tens of thousands offering to host refugee families in their homes for many months. But that spirit rarely persists; after the honeymoon, people tend to become more pessimistic and self-protective, and move on.

So, the slowing sense of solidarity and collective response we saw some months into the pandemic was entirely normal.

But there was at least one potential major accelerant to the process. The end of the clap had coincided with the "Dominic Cummings affair", the news that the Prime Minister's most senior adviser had travelled to a small town in North East England for unexplained reasons. These actions were seemingly a blatant breach of lockdown rules. Previously, less high-profile individuals involved in the government's response to Covid had committed breaches. They included the epidemiologist Professor Niall Ferguson, responsible for some of the most influential initial pandemic modelling, and Catherine Calderwood, the Scottish chief medical officer. They had lost their jobs. But, this time, the situation was more serious as the behaviour of the Prime Minister's chief advisor and the architect of many aspects of the pandemic response contradicted the nightly order to "Stay at home, Save the NHS, Save lives" given by the Prime Minister and senior medics. Not only was he a more significant figure in the Covid response than the previous two resignees, but he was backed by the Prime Minister and stayed in post.

There was a fear that this would undermine the sense of collective purpose that had characterised the pandemic to date, especially as it was conveyed in the popular press as being "One rule for us, one rule for them."

Trust really matters in a pandemic. Given that (as discussed) the measures people are being asked to take are primarily designed to protect strangers rather than themselves or loved ones, if people feel others can't be trusted, they are less likely to make the sacrifices themselves. Why should they? An academic study across ten countries during the pandemic showed that where trust fell, so did compliance.[27] In the UK, trust fell significantly from the early days of the pandemic as the months progressed.

---

[27] Francesco Sarracino, Talita Greyling, Kelsey J. O'Connor, Chiara Peroni, Stephanie Rossouw, Trust predicts compliance with COVID-19 containment policies: Evidence from ten countries using big data, Economics & Human Biology, Volume 54, 2024.

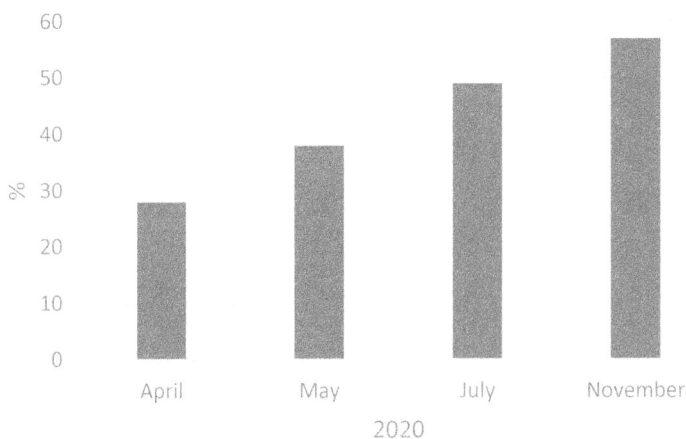

Percentage who trust government "not very much" or "not at all" to control the spread of Coronavirus, year 2020. Source: Bobby Duffy, King's College London.[28]

So, in September 2020, as we started to see cases rising again, and with the knowledge that a consistent increase through the autumn would leave us potentially seriously exposed in winter, it felt hard to mobilise people once more. It also felt that we had lost one of the critical messages of the pandemic, that our individual behaviours were not about the risks we chose to take for ourselves, but the steps we were willing to take to protect others.

As debates would unfold over the coming months, from whether to obey social distancing rules to face coverings, people would often say they were willing to 'take the risk', not recognising that it was not about their personal risk tolerance towards getting Covid, but the risks we collectively posed to each other as potential transmitters.

---

[28] https://www.kcl.ac.uk/policy-institute/assets/the-handling-of-the-coronavirus-crisis.pdf

Government messaging seemed to shift, too. Perhaps this was connected to the breakdown in trust following the Cummings affair. It simply didn't make sense for senior government politicians to talk about collective responsibility all the time now, as it would merely highlight apparent hypocrisy. It felt like they backed away from the messaging of collective effort and focused increasingly on compliance around individual behaviours. Not only did the police have powers if people flouted Covid regulations, but local authorities were handed funds for Covid marshals to patrol high footfall areas and remind people of the rules.

This links to a phenomenon that has previously been recognised in public health policy, called "lifestyle drift". This concept holds that – although evidence suggests health inequalities are caused by the broader social and environmental conditions of people's lives – it is easier for policymakers to focus on individual behaviours; behaviours such as how can we help people make better choices about eating, smoking, or drinking, rather than getting to the root causes of obesity or the reasons people from poorer backgrounds are more likely to smoke. Placing the onus on individual choices – rather than the conditions in which they arise – is less likely to be effective but allows policymakers to redirect blame from ineffective policymaking to irresponsible citizens.

While the national mood definitely made things harder, we were still trying to establish that strong sense of communal purpose locally. I was optimistic that the Champions programme we had begun to establish in the early summer was now gaining momentum, both locally and (to our surprise) nationally. In Newham, we had hundreds of participants, and large numbers joined weekly calls. We regularly shared the work nationally and supported many other authorities in establishing equivalent schemes. It gave me a vehicle for trying to engender feelings of community and solidarity in an ongoing way in our response. The Champions' conversations were inspiring. Every time I joined an evening Zoom call, it left me with a greater sense of optimism and hope that *by working together* we could navigate the next phase of the pandemic.

These Zoom calls would carry on throughout the whole pandemic. Over time, they got harder to mobilise, and it became tougher to engage large numbers. After all, our lives moved on to other things. Unity is tricky to build and maintain outside the burning platform of a national crisis, particularly without the support and communication tools that a national government has. However, the collective sense of purpose at many moments of the pandemic were a sign of the ability to mobilise solidarity locally, around common purpose. It may be harder in normal times, but the rewards definitely make it worth trying.

Chapter 14
The Slow-Motion Car Crash

As September 2020 arrived, alongside schools returning to some degree of normality, there was widespread encouragement from the government for people to get on with aspects of everyday life. This included the suggestion that office workers should return to work.

A parody of the government's pandemic slogan circulated on social media. Instead of "Stay at home, Save the NHS, Save Lives", the mantra had become "Leave home, forget the NHS, Save Pret" (the ubiquitous city centre sandwich seller). There was a sense that the political priority had shifted from managing the risk of Covid to getting the economy going again. While there were many advocates for greater levels of social restriction, fresh on the heels of "Eat Out to Help Out", the government was not convinced of the need for further restrictive measures.

Throughout September and October 2020, the number of Covid cases rose steadily. On the one hand, things felt manageable; health services were coping ok, although only if one disregarded the ever-increasing backlog of non-Covid health needs (they were being deprioritised with incredibly significant short- and long-term effects). On the other hand, the general acceptance of this level of infection and sickness without vaccination or evidence-based treatments felt problematic.

Of course, there were still lots of restrictions in place. For all the attempts at normality, life clearly didn't remotely resemble our pre-pandemic existence, and with the ongoing wait for news from vaccine trials, the trajectory of the pandemic remained highly uncertain. The rising infection rates, in particular, were creating concern about how the

NHS would manage over the winter period, when health services typically struggle even at the best of times.

With rates rising steadily, after the half-term school break in October 2020, the government announced a "circuit breaker" – a four-week lockdown to try to curtail further growth. Many had been arguing for this for weeks, but the government had resisted, trying to balance the different needs of society. As the Prime Minister, Boris Johnson, said when announcing the new measures:

"This is a constant struggle and balance that any government has to make between lives and livelihoods, and lives must come first, but we have to be mindful of the scarring, the long-term economic impact of the measures."

In Newham, the impact of the new measures was to slow the rate of growth in infections, but in absolute terms, the number of new infections continued to rise. Scrutinising my data, I wondered how cases were continuing to grow when so many restrictions were in place; even with Newham's particular vulnerabilities, it didn't make sense.

Then, in early December 2020, something unimaginable happened.

Despite the many restrictions, the number of cases in East London suddenly went from steadily rising to exploding. First, this happened in outer London (the London boroughs of Havering & Barking and Dagenham), but it soon followed into Newham and the neighbouring boroughs as well. What was going on? Nothing had specifically changed in the restrictions to have such a dramatic effect. Nothing was going on specifically in North East London, either (well, that we were aware of), despite attempts by some – largely on social media – to claim that this was a behavioural issue of non-compliance (an old East London trope, revived with racist undertones). I was worried.

The boroughs were called to an urgent meeting by senior London leaders. Policymakers, both nationally and across London, were concerned. The restrictions that had been in force from the beginning of November had been intended to ensure the NHS could manage in winter and that, after such a challenging year, people could celebrate Christmas with some semblance of normality. In turn, it was hoped that businesses would be able to reap the benefit of the festive trade, something that was important to the economy.

At this point in the pandemic, there were different levels of restrictions across the country, based on the local perceived level of risk. We were told that we had to try to keep levels down and stop the spread to other parts of the city, or we risked pushing London into a higher level of restrictions. This was alarming. Was there really a belief that *local* action – in a huge, mobile, interconnected city such as London – could halt the rapid spread of a respiratory virus?

Epidemiologists often use "doubling time" as a way of understanding and communicating the relative speed of an infection spreading over a given period. When the case rate took off in early December, the doubling went from over a month to doubling in a week. Visually, it is even more impactful. We can compare the actual data we saw to what would have happened if case numbers had continued to grow at the same rate.

The figure below shows the dramatic difference between a hypothetical scenario of a steady state and what we actually saw. Given that – pre-vaccination – case numbers translated fairly reliably into a proportion of hospital admissions, a percentage then converted into numbers in intensive care, and a further proportion into deaths, this rate of growth was frankly terrifying.

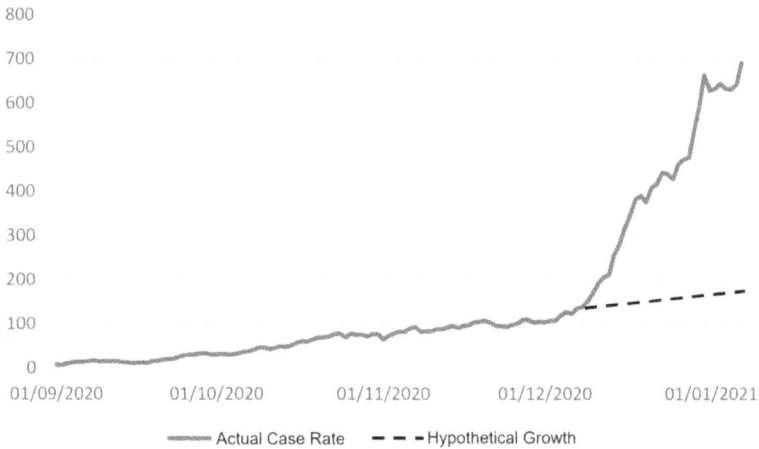

*Average actual and modelled number of daily cases in Newham,
1 September 2020 - 6 January 2021.*

It's worth going back a few months here. In the summer following the first wave, attention had turned to preparedness for the rest of the pandemic. One aspect of this was a discussion about the approaches and plans that local areas needed to put in place to complement national action. Each local authority, alongside others such as the NHS, schools, and other local organisations, was required to pull together a Local Outbreak Management Plan, setting out the steps they would take in response to an escalation of cases. We wrote what I considered to be a decent plan, drawing on the range of tools we had, with thoughtful sections on community engagement, good collaboration with our local partners, utilising local politicians, and trigger points for further escalation.

However, I always worried whether these plans would be meaningful in real-world Covid situations. Local or community outbreak management is typically applicable when an infection is circulating in a relatively defined population: a geographical area, a neighbourhood, or amongst a particularly interconnected community, such as the MPox outbreak among men who have sex with men (MSM), which occurred in summer 2022, or meningitis in a particular student population.

But Covid was different, and London was different still. Covid is a respiratory virus that transmits incredibly easily between people. Combined with the highly interconnected, kinetic world of big cities like London, it felt legitimate to ask whether the virus could really be contained to a specific locality in this context.

In metropolitan urban areas, my "community" isn't bounded by the streets I live in; I work on the other side of the city from where I live, with colleagues spread across the wider South East region of England. Many of my friends are also spread out. Moreover, the large Tesco where I shop has a significant catchment area used by people from many neighbourhoods. For others, a range of convening points, such as places of worship or their children's schools or even their favourite hairdressers, bring them into close contact with people from other parts of the city. Perhaps in smaller, more bounded places like Leicester – where the first geographically-focused concern emerged from the aftermath of the first wave – local outbreak management was more realistic. While Leicester has almost exactly the population size as Newham, the latter is just one of 32 interconnected London boroughs, all surrounded by the dense, interlinked hinterland of the Home Counties.

As we developed our outbreak plan, we also tried to work out our trigger points when we would escalate to additional measures. But I felt that a more likely scenario for the coming months was a city-wide or sub-regional "rising tide" rather than a single borough spike in cases. In other words, I foresaw a growing number of cases over a wide area rather than a specific increase in a small, defined locality without corresponding rises elsewhere. We would see certain schools with large outbreaks, but they wouldn't necessarily be next door to each other; they would be spread around the wider area, and beyond that, it would be hard to pinpoint particular places.

These different scenarios mattered to our strategic planning. If you believed that local outbreak management could work against a localised increase of Covid cases in one part of a metropolitan area, such as London, then it made sense to give it significant focus. Why invest time and resources, or inflict restrictions with their social and economic consequences, on other unaffected areas if you can control the virus in one part of the city? But conversely, if you believe that a spike in cases in one part of the city is merely an early warning of what is about to come, and that – without wider action – the infection is inevitably going to reach other parts of the city, then a predominantly local focus without a wider regional or national response is simply going to invite further spread.

This takes us back to December 2020. The East London boroughs were getting together with their outbreak management plans, and had been tasked with trying to stop the march of Covid across the city, ruining Christmas for everyone else. It never felt realistic, though. We had a couple of additional tools we could use, such as mobile testing units, which could be placed on our high streets and encourage people without symptoms to come test in order to limit asymptomatic transmission. We also had the opportunity to develop a network of test sites using the new rapid Lateral Flow Tests (LFT). Over time, they would become as commonplace for people as their wallets and mobile phones, but they were brand new at that point.

The LFTs had just been piloted in Liverpool in November 2020 with a huge mobilisation that aimed to control a rising tide in the city. In Liverpool, the army had come out in large numbers, and they essentially tried to test the whole metropolis. In the first two weeks, over 150,000 tests were conducted, equating to nearly one in every three city residents. It was early days, but there was some hope that this 'whole population approach' to identifying the asymptomatic carriage of Covid had managed to turn around the situation in the city.

There were two major differences in North East London, the first of which I could see clearly from the start. The level of mobilisation being proposed in North East London was a small fraction of what was done in Liverpool. This was a population of two million – four times that of Liverpool – but there was no army involvement or huge deployment of a testing workforce from elsewhere. We were given a handful of mobile testing units and the promise of money to create systems for rapid testing. The former would reach small numbers, take weeks to organise, and still be far smaller than the Liverpool approach.

The second difference was invisible to the human eye and only became apparent some days later. On the 14th of December, Matt Hancock, the Secretary of State for Health, announced that Public Health England laboratories had identified a new genetic variant of Covid-19 – B117. Known in the UK as the *Kent* variant, because of the county where it was initially identified, this strain was known internationally as the UK variant. The first sample had been taken nearly two months earlier and had slowly spread through the southern English county across the autumn. Perhaps the comparative population sparsity in the "Garden of England", as Kent is known, and the different demographic characteristics it had in comparison to metropolitan London, hid the impact of B117, but by the time it arrived at scale in North East London, it started to take off. Indeed, it crowded out the original or "wild-type" strain rapidly.

The social restrictions that had been perfectly sufficient to maintain or slow the rate of growth were no longer adequate. This helped explain why rates had continued to rise through the November lockdown, despite significant curbs in place. Daily, I sat looking at my data, waiting, hoping that the actions we were taking, combined with national restrictions, would turn the tide, but they didn't.

As the Covid cases rose exponentially, I was getting increasingly vexed. The number of infections was piling higher than anything we had seen before, suggesting an extraordinary health crisis around New Year and very significant loss of life. Yet the government seemed committed to Christmas this year. I was incredulous.

Surely a normal Christmas could wait? After all, people in Newham had forgone their Eid and Diwali celebrations. But more importantly, we had just begun the vaccination programme. This remarkable effort by vaccine scientists and pharmaceutical production to get Covid vaccines ready and at scale in just months had achieved what few thought possible (the next chapter will focus on this in more detail). But the impact of not introducing restrictions at this point meant that many people would die. Logically, if we introduced restrictions at this point, they would soon be vaccinated, and they would survive.

Throughout the pandemic, I recognised the incredibly tough decisions that politicians and their advisors faced. Often, the choice was between the least bad option(s), and there were always multiple factors to consider. Ultimately, things would boil down to questions of judgment; there were no right answers.

I also tried, the whole way through, to take a rounded view of risk and impact, considering social and economic effects, mental health, education, and other factors, as well as infection control. These were equally important areas that needed to be considered. I accepted that these uncertainties and complexities meant that even the most rational of people might often disagree on the right approach. However, on this one, I was clear: with this level of risk, and mass vaccination *around the corner*, we needed to act faster.

One small incident at this time showed the complexity of decision-making. Although it was mid-winter, a planned running event in my area was set to go ahead. To me, it ticked many positive boxes: it was outside, the organisers had worked to limit the number of runners, there would be no standing around and chatting, it was purposeful, social, and physically active. Given all the organisers' work, and compared to many, many things, it was safe. But others had heard about the event and asked me to withdraw my support. My initial reaction was not to; the event was legal and relatively safe, and not far away was an open indoor shopping centre where huge crowds were gathering to do their pre-Christmas shopping.

We had limited powers with the shopping centre, but the inconsistency and disproportionality of closing down the run felt deeply uncomfortable. I continued to come under pressure from different local and city partners about how this looked – the hospital was under the most intense pressure with a critical incident on the verge of being declared, and we were allowing a fun run to go ahead? Against my stronger instincts, I bowed to the voices of those who wanted it not to happen. I understood what they were going through, even if I instinctively disagreed with the outcome. So, a few runners were prevented from being active outside while thousands shopped indoors nearby.

Eventually, the government put London into lockdown, but it was too late to limit the damage, which now exceeded what we had seen in the first Covid wave. Lockdown would follow shortly for the country as a whole, and schools closed once more. By the time restrictions came, the Kent variant had spread widely.

This was – without doubt – my lowest point in the pandemic. In the first wave, I, like many, was on the steepest of learning curves. Yes, I felt that lockdown should have begun a week earlier, and I believe that would have saved many lives, but the speed of events, the uncertainty of the moment, and the overwhelming novelty of the challenge were unmatched.

This *was* different.

December 2020 was, for me, like watching a slow-motion car crash. This time, I understood what was going on. I had a strong sense of what I believed needed to happen. I felt a deep responsibility to the community where I worked, particularly with what they had been through during the first wave, yet I felt powerless to effect the necessary change. The concept of moral injury made even more sense to me now.

Over the course of the second wave, from November 2020 to February 2021, there were over 80,000 Covid deaths in the UK.

Each day, I would check the data to see signs of the tide turning, looking at my tables of newly reported cases for glimmers of hope. For days, the numbers only got worse.

Many people talk of that period as particularly hard. It was yet another long lockdown, and our collective resilience was running low. Solidarity and trust had fallen and it was winter. The first lockdown – when the enormous challenges and fear were partially mitigated by novelty and sunshine – had been replaced by cold. It was hard.

For us, as a family, we had one particular ray of sunshine: our son's bar mitzvah, the Jewish coming of age celebration at age 13, normally celebrated and surrounded by community, family, and friends in a synagogue and at a party with dancing. It was consigned to Zoom. But we embraced it, planning a special occasion, and while it wasn't what anyone would have chosen, it gave us a joyous focus in this otherwise grim period. The extent of my son's in-person social interactions was a series of two-person walks with his closest friends one snowy Sunday, wrapped up warm and clutching hot chocolate. A quintessential pandemic experience. We appreciated what small and simple pleasures we could.

On January 6th 2021, over 1,000 new cases were reported in a single day, nearly ten times the number of cases reported five weeks earlier. That was the peak. From then on, cases started to drop significantly, and once again, we could turn from despair to hope: the belief that there was a way to steer ourselves out of this. What's more, attention would now focus on the really big opportunity and challenge we faced: vaccination.

Chapter 15
Vaccinating Newham

For so many months, we had lived with unprecedented uncertainty. Although the pandemic had ebbed and flowed, without an effective, safe vaccine available, there was little prospect of life truly returning to normal.

We learned that the normal rulebook had been ripped up, and that vaccine scientists and pharmaceutical companies were working at unimaginable speed with the support of governments to get population-ready vaccines developed, tested, and manufactured. As early as May 2020, participants were being given initial vaccine doses as part of the development programme. On the 2nd of December 2020, less than a year into the pandemic, the Medicines and Healthcare products Regulatory Agency (MHRA) approved the Pfizer vaccine for use in the UK. (A few weeks later, the Oxford/AstraZeneca vaccine was also approved.) On the 8th of December, Margaret Keenan, a 90-year-old in Coventry, became the first recipient.

Over the next year, we would go on a remarkable journey to ensure the vaccines reached our population in Newham. As much as I had learned about public health in my career, and through the pandemic to date, the vaccine programme would teach me so much about my work and the place I worked. It was a creative and thoughtful time, a period that encompassed some deep frustrations but also enormous highs.

The concept of vaccine hesitancy was much discussed throughout the country as political and health leaders and media alike tried to make sense of differing vaccination rates in different areas and among different demographic slices of the population (we will return to explore this). The community where I lived (as opposed to worked) was anything but "vaccine hesitant". Indeed, we could be reasonably described as being "vaccine eager"! People would wait with great anticipation for the first chance to get vaccinated, share on WhatsApp if they knew of spare vaccine vials at a particular GP or pharmacy that would go to people even if they weren't age-eligible, and who would talk proudly about which vaccine they had been given (Pfizer, AstraZeneca, or Moderna). Of course, some parts of Newham were like this, and others were not.

But was it vaccine hesitance or something more multifaceted and complex that slowed uptake? Six months into the vaccine programme, we held an event on Zoom where people shared their vaccine stories, including what had caused them (or a friend or family member) to take the vaccine.

We heard about the challenges the adult children of older migrant parents faced. Where language barriers, digital access, or basic cultural navigation meant that invitation letters would have gone unread if supportive children had not opened the post, made appointments, and escorted their parents to the vaccination centres. We heard of imams and priests who had convinced people about the importance of the vaccine, combatting doubts circulating within people's Facebook streams. We heard of persuasive and encouraging GPs who, with great tenacity, had supported people who were very unsure. And we bore witness to friends who had given other friends the confidence they needed when they were otherwise fearful. There were many other examples.

We began to talk about how "it takes a village to vaccinate a community", when so many barriers can get in the way of straightforward take-up.

Our work on vaccination had started early. While the Covid Champions were often viewed as a conduit to cascade messages across the community, they were equally important

– to us – as a way of hearing the concerns of our residents. As the positive stories of vaccines having excellent results in trials started to be reported, but before any approvals (let alone delivery) had begun, our Champions were telling us about vaccine anxiety and the work that needed to be done locally. We needed to get people on board.

We started a series of community conversations, even before we knew very much, drawing on the same approach we had used with our Covid Champions throughout the pandemic. Our principles were: to share our collective expertise with residents, to ensure they were informed, to be honest about what we knew and didn't know (a lot in the early stages), to be transparent about our opinions and non-judgmental about theirs, and to try to answer every question they had.

We put together a great team, alongside our public health unit, that would work on these community events for over a year. It included local GPs Dr Muhammad Naqvi and Dr Vaishali Ashar, a local consultant on sexual health and HIV Medicine, Dr Vanessa Apea, Professor Winston Morgan, an immensely knowledgeable and thoughtful toxicologist from the University of East London with a particular interest in vaccination uptake among ethnic minorities, as well as myself and other colleagues from the NHS.

We would invite others, too, and found that people were incredibly willing to help. A friend, Dr Marianne Cunnington, a vaccine epidemiologist and an expert on vaccine safety who was working for a pharmaceutical company, even came along for one session to share her knowledge and perspectives. Indeed, her visit left us with greater insight to pass on to the community. At times, our local politicians joined us as well, to lead by example. Anne Pordes-Bowers, our Covid Champions lead, expertly led these sessions, as ever.

These community conversations helped build up the knowledge of those who attended. Crucially, they established a culture of transparency and trust as well. The number we reached through these sessions was small compared to Newham's population of over 350,000, and it was hard to measure the wider impact. However, I believe it set a tone in the borough where professionals and residents could talk about the vaccine, and that stood us well. That spirit pervaded as we built out the networks of vaccine champions and community sites.

As I participated in these discussions, hearing the perspectives of different professionals and the wide and varied insights and views of community members, the idea of vaccine hesitancy made increasing sense to me. When almost all of us go for a medical appointment and agree to some form of medical intervention, we engage in a trust process. That is inevitable as there is a huge knowledge asymmetry between us, as patients, and doctors. This situation, of course, applied to the vaccine. I don't really know what is in the vaccine and have only a superficial understanding of the biochemical process involved. Neither have I reviewed the safety data that bodies like the Medicine and Healthcare products Regulatory Agency have issued, nor, even with my public health training, would I understand them with any depth even if I did. Instead, I trust.

I trust the people and the processes, and my life has largely taught me that believing in these people and these processes has served me well. If society's institutions had let me down at points in my life – and, in particular, if medical institutions had acted in ways which betrayed that trust – would I feel the same about any intervention?

As far as the vaccine was concerned, the speed of its development was bound to create doubts. Later, when the vaccine became available for younger age groups, many individuals wondered – given the limited impact of Covid on younger people and rare negative impact – whether it was worth having. It made me wonder how many of my peers, so eager to return to international travel, when you needed the vaccine to enter most countries, would have been as quick to take up the vaccine if they hadn't been so keen to go abroad.

Around eight months after being alerted that the Excel Centre would be turned into the first Nightingale Hospital, I received another call telling me that it was about to be converted into a mass vaccination centre, delivering thousands of vaccines per day. In many ways, the symbolism was a powerfully optimistic one. The same setting that was an emergency field hospital to cope with thousands of people who needed intensive care but couldn't be served by our standard hospitals (and where, in reality, many people would likely have died) would now be a place of salvation where people could come to be protected. But I couldn't focus on that symbolism. What seemed obvious to me was that local people wouldn't come.

The reason for this can be hard to explain and sometimes difficult to understand.

My gut feeling could be best explained by a story I heard many years earlier in my career. My wife had known a youth worker based on a housing estate in Gospel Oak, a neighbourhood in inner North London. The teenage boys he worked with were tough and not engaged with school, but he connected with them as great youth workers do. He discovered they were all huge football fans and, in particular, devoted to the local team… Arsenal. One day, he managed to secure tickets for all of them for a match. He arranged to meet the boys at Arsenal underground station, almost opposite the old Highbury ground where they played their matches in those days. He waited and waited, but they never came. He was worried. Had something happened to one of them? Had they got in a fight on the way? He eventually gave up and made his way back to the estate – where the boys lived – and found them hanging out in the same spot where they always were. What had happened, he asked. Why did they not come to meet him for the match? They replied that they didn't know how to get there and were too embarrassed to ask. The ground of the team they supported with passion and love was only two miles away, but those two miles were too far for them.

I saw the parallels with some parts of Newham's community and the planned mass vaccination centre, and we fed back to the powers-that-be that we didn't think this site – a vast anonymous exhibition centre in a relatively inaccessible part of the borough – was a good idea. To get high vaccine take-up, we needed to be very local, in places that people knew and trusted and could access easily. Ideally, this would mean local GP practices or pharmacies, but potentially also leisure centres, community centres, or places of worship. Many had halls that could serve as effective clinics. Initially, we were told no… this was not the plan.

It was deeply frustrating. We knew our communities. We had learned much over the years, but even more through the previous months of the pandemic. We would speak to people in the NHS who largely agreed with us, but it was impossible to find people in the immense bureaucracy with whom we could have a proper conversation about the plan.

The vaccine programme started slowly in Newham. That was always going to be the case. We had a small older population, and the beginning of the programme was focused on older people and frontline health and care workers. We had argued that in areas with large minority populations, the age should be lower for the start of the programme because all of the evidence showed a disproportionate impact at a young age in minority groups with underlying health conditions. However, that argument failed to gain traction. So, we built our engagement programme, developing what we called our Supportive Conversations approach – an informative but non-judgmental and evidence-based way of spreading information across all kinds of settings in the borough, from places of worship to care homes and schools. Our Community Champions and elected councillors helped us build connections with different communities, which widened our outreach opportunities. For example, local councillors brokered access to a huge online Nigerian evangelical church, where we could do question and answer sessions or hold much more intimate in-person gatherings with our care staff.

As the weeks moved on and the age groups eligible for the vaccine became younger, it became evident that we needed to work to get the NHS to change tack; many NHS colleagues agreed. The limited number of GP and pharmacy sites alongside mass vaccination centres at the Excel Centre and the Westfield shopping complex would just not get the job done. We needed considerably more capacity for vaccinations outside the large centres. It was still early in the programme, late January 2021, but I felt we were at risk of drifting.

One of my amazing team members during the pandemic was a young, early-career public health professional called Yszi Hawkins. She was one of those people you could always turn to when you just needed something doing, and she had worked tirelessly over the previous 12 months. She was having much-needed time off, but I was getting desperate, and I knew she was the person for this job. I messaged her and asked if I could interrupt her leave for a brief conversation. We spoke about the need for a huge immunisation outreach programme focusing on the places of worship across the borough: mosques, Sikh gurdwaras, Hindu temples, and churches connecting to different parts of our multi-ethnic communities. She was generous as ever and up for the challenge. When Yszi returned from leave, she would deprioritise everything else and focus on this. Over the next year, she did a phenomenal job.

We started by inviting faith communities to a meeting where we would explain what we wanted to do and why, what we would need from them regarding space and facilities, and to answer any questions. We were overwhelmed by the response. Over 40 communities turned up for the meeting.

Far from being symbols of vaccine hesitancy, these community leaders had seen the impact of Covid first-hand; they had officiated at funerals, consoled mourners, lost dedicated members of their congregations and communities, and wanted to help. In fact, there was much more enthusiasm than we could support. We were limited by issues such as vaccine supply, storage, and trained vaccinators, but working with our local NHS colleagues – who ultimately brought great flexibility and commitment to this way of working – we built as ambitious a plan as we could.

Over the many months that followed, we delivered tens of thousands of doses to our outreach clinics, which grew from the faith groups to community centres, shopping centre car parks, sheltered housing, high streets and, ultimately, a major clinic in one of our leisure centres in East Ham in the heart of Newham. In the end, we would use well over 50 outreach sites across the borough. Time and again, we could see the benefit of holding these clinics in these hyper-local, walkable, and trusted venues for our population. The venues themselves gave everything voluntarily in terms of space and volunteers' time. They received no financial benefit or even financial support; it was the community in action, the state and community working hand in hand, not on a transactional basis but out of common purpose.

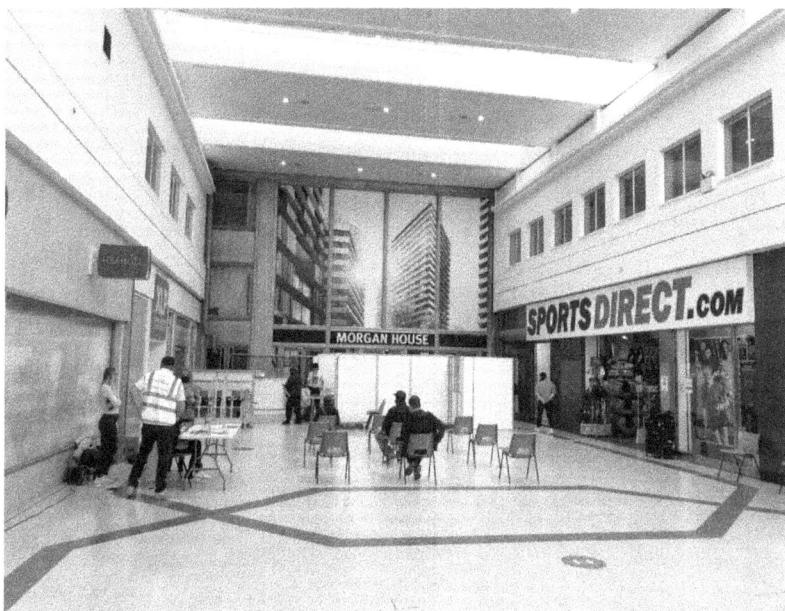

Covid vaccine clinic in Stratford Shopping Mall.

As the months went on, summer 2021 drew closer, and we started to reach the younger cohorts in the adult vaccination programme. In Newham, most adults are between 18 and 40, so the population as a whole would remain relatively unvaccinated until this group of residents was eligible.

The first weekend that under-30s were eligible for the vaccine was a summer scorcher. We had extensively advertised a big two-day immunisation weekend at our leisure centre in East Ham, and organised a well-staffed clinic, hoping for decent numbers. I had wanted to organise music and entertainment, but all we managed to provide was bottled water and a few gazebos. I cycled down on the Saturday morning to see how it was going, and as I reached the centre, I was utterly astonished. The queue of Newham's young people, evidently from all of the communities in the borough, snaked back and forth and around the block. Young people waited in the heat, many for over three hours, for their vaccine. The mood and spirit were totally positive, with thousands of "vaccine-eager" young adults waiting patiently for their turn; no complaints, just playing their part in our collective effort. The vaccinators I spoke to said that no one was cross for having to wait, and most people just offered their profuse thanks to those working all day in the heat to protect them and their community. Over two days, at that site alone, we vaccinated more than 4,000 young adults.

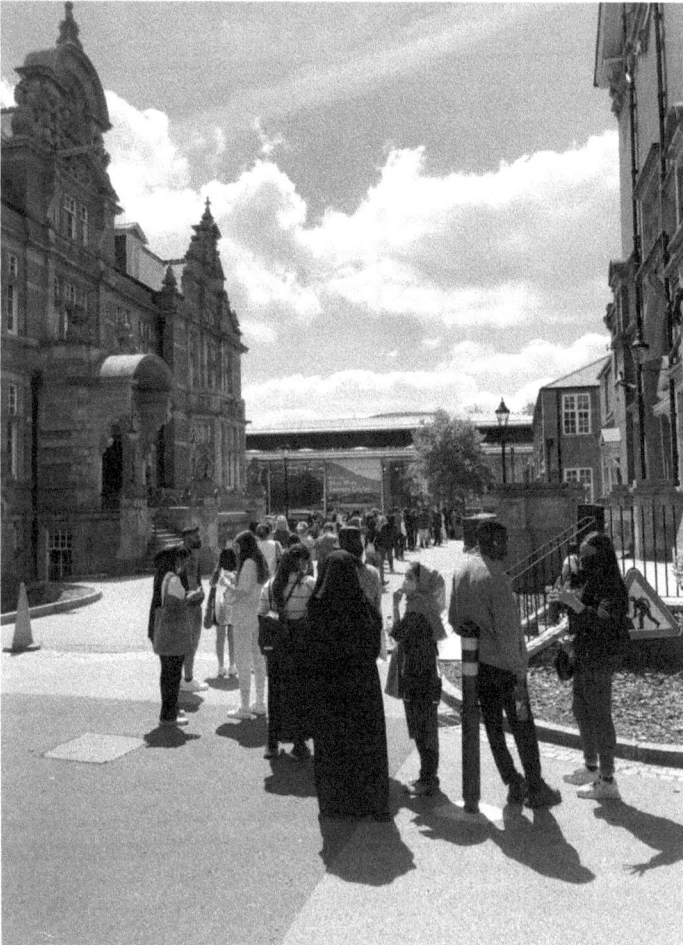

Young adults queuing for up to three hours for their Covid vaccine,
East Ham, Summer 2021.

Throughout the vaccination programme, we worked as if we were a software development team using processes akin to agile, scrum, and sprints to constantly evolve our approaches, test new models, and adapt our activities based on the evidence and insight we received. We thought deeply about how to reach more people with the Covid vaccine and tested many different approaches, including outreach work, multigenerational housing pilots, the funding of tiny grassroots community groups, and even a schools vaccine poster competition.

One of the winning posters in the Newham Schools vaccine competition; by Nawailah Makardam in the 12-18 age category from Plashet School.

We thought a lot about an approach articulated by SAGE, the government's Scientific Advisory Group for Emergencies. They drew on a WHO approach, a 3Cs model – Convenience, Complacency, Confidence – based on evidence and behavioural insight that explained lower vaccine take-up to help develop strategies to combat it. From our own experience and insight in Newham, we began to reframe this to talk about Accessibility, Relevance, and Trust (ART). We saw the 3Cs as focusing on how people not taking up vaccines needed to change, rather than understanding the very real barriers that existed to take up (which we, as policymakers and service providers, needed to address).

So, in our formulation, "Accessibility" more than "Convenience" describes the experience of people who:

- are housebound and unable to access clinic-based services

- have inflexible employment or caring requirements

- lack digital access, or who may not receive information or be able to make bookings online

- have limited English or social capital and struggle to navigate the system

"Relevance" more than "Complacency" describes the experience of people who, for example, face competing priorities, where the importance of a particular intervention – such as testing, isolating, or vaccination – is weighed against other needs, such as concern over maintaining employment or losing wages.

"Trust" more than "Confidence" describes what is required to accept certain messages, services, and interventions. Most of us face some imbalance of expertise and information when offered health advice and medical intervention. While many of us have good reasons to trust this advice, the lived experiences of others may make them more fearful, influenced by damaging personal and/or collective histories, alongside competing voices championing alternative narratives. Low trust connects closely to stigma, being judged, or perceiving that we will be negatively assessed for an aspect of ourselves, our beliefs, or behaviours.

As a public health team in Newham, the more we've reflected since, the more we've come to think these questions are deeply relevant to *all public services*, and we intend to keep exploring them.

How did we do overall? With such a young, diverse, mobile population, the barriers to vaccination take-up would always be significant. We know we reached many thousands through our community vaccination clinics, although – strangely enough – it's hard to tell exactly how much of our population we reached. You would think the basic function of local governance is to know how many people live in your area. Throughout the pandemic, we were regularly towards the bottom of the league tables for vaccination rate as the numbers the NHS used for our population denominator had 60-70,000 more people than the census estimated for our population. This vast discrepancy mostly occurred in the 18-40 age group, the bulk of Newham's population. I realised that we had vaccinated more people than were on the electoral register, and when the 2021 census results were released, this difference stood out once again. Throughout much of the pandemic, I told myself not to worry about the discrepancy; my job was to vaccinate as many people as we could – I couldn't control this difference. But it does matter.

It matters because it tells you how much effort you need to continue putting into any single issue at the expense of others. If we're chasing shadows, we would be better off putting our limited resources into the many other health challenges that exist.

But it also matters because the numbers inform a perception of a place. Is Newham a place full of vaccine-hesitant people, or one that pulled together remarkably well? Journalists often asked me about vaccine hesitancy in the borough, and I always explained the challenges using numbers. While there were differences in take-up for different ethnic groups, even with the inflated denominators, we know that most people from all backgrounds got vaccinated.

Throughout the vaccination programme, I saw very real differences between the community where I lived and where I worked. I knew that vaccine take-up would be more straightforward in the former than the latter. But I also learned that these barriers were not as great as often assumed, and that they were surmountable with thought, effort, and collaboration, meaning there would be lessons from this experience that went well beyond the pandemic.

Chapter 16

Malawi and Omicron – A Global Personal Perspective

Throughout 2021, life began to resemble something a bit more normal. Over the summer, restrictions on social gatherings had largely ended, and – despite fairly ubiquitous face masks and vaccine passports – the end of the pandemic felt very much in touching distance. The vaccine programme was a huge success, and the numbers in hospital from Covid had plummeted alongside deaths from the disease. The only potential uncertainty on the horizon was from new variants. Might there emerge a new Covid strain that was vaccine-resistant, halting our collective progress to normality?

In November 2021, Malawi in South East Africa came off the UK's red list for travel, allowing people from the UK to visit the country without needing to quarantine on their return home. It was news I had been longing for. A very close friend, Sydney Simumba, was in the end stages of cancer, following diagnosis in late 2019. I wanted to spend some final moments with him.

I had known Sydney for 17 years. A chance encounter with Sydney and two other young Malawian teachers, John Chaula and Feston Singoyi, on my honeymoon had led to a lasting friendship and partnership and the founding of a UK charity called Masambiro UK (www.masambiro.org.uk). Amongst other projects, the charity led to the creation of Kunyanja Secondary School, which, to date, has supported more than 12,000 children in education and sent hundreds to university. Sydney was its inspirational headteacher. Alongside my work, this has been a very significant part of my adult life.

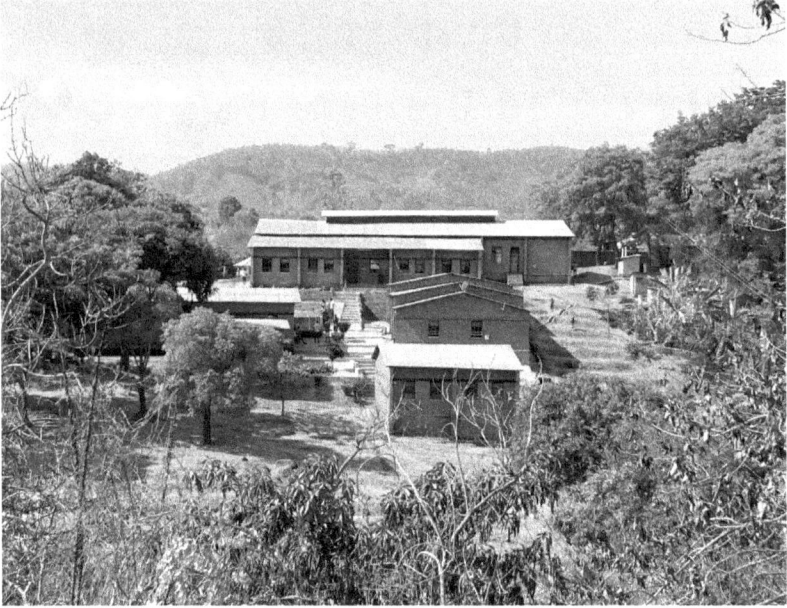

Kunyanja Secondary School in Nkhata Bay, Malawi.

My relationship with Malawi over this time has given me new and different perspectives on the health challenges faced in different parts of the world. Malawi is an extremely poor country with a GDP of $625 per capita (compared to over $40,000 in the UK). I've been many times over the years; I love the country and feel very comfortable there. But every time I arrive, I am still thrown by the scale of the differences between the digital, urban, affluent society that I experience as entirely normal, and the agricultural, rural society of everyday life in Malawi. The material differences are just immense. Many of the children at the school live in families who are subsistence farmers. The culture expects that anyone who earns a salary to pay for as many of their extended family to go to school as they can afford.

The health challenges Malawians face are enormous.

When our work in Malawi began, Southern Africa was still in the midst of its enormous HIV/AIDS challenge. Anti-retroviral drugs, although widely available in more prosperous countries, remained scarce. Some years later, John Chaula, one of the three teachers we began to work with in 2004, during the early years of the school, sadly passed away from AIDS.

Malawi also faces countless everyday challenges from malaria, which is a leading cause of death, alongside public health issues like a lack of clean water (there have been cholera outbreaks in recent years), and the absence of very basic healthcare. For example, at the school for deaf children in Bandawe, where we built a connection, many of the students had been left without hearing because of an inability to treat simple childhood ear infections that in the UK would be treated with uncomplicated and inexpensive antibiotics.

When Sydney contacted me to tell of his likely cancer diagnosis in November 2019, his assumption was that he would go home to his village to die. Without even much basic primary healthcare available in Malawi, more specialist treatments – as required for cancers – are beyond the capabilities of the country and most citizens. When Sydney was diagnosed, there was one oncologist in Malawi, a country of 20 million people and no radiotherapy. We arranged to support Sydney in going to South Africa for diagnosis and treatment, and while he was there, the pandemic began. Sadly, the treatment was too late, and his diagnosis was terminal. Eventually, despite lockdowns, he managed to get an evacuation bus from Cape Town back to Malawi in late spring of 2020.

Sydney was an incredible man, full of ambition. Despite coming home with the awful news, he was desperate to help his community navigate the challenges of Covid. But what did this mean? In the first wave of the pandemic in the UK, we had heard stories of TV medical dramas *Holby City* and

Casualty donating actual working ventilators to the NHS when many African countries had few or even none. Combatting Covid in Malawi wasn't about access to intensive care in hospital, but trying to do the basics of limiting the spread of infection. Sydney and Feston asked for money from our charity for buckets and soap and printed informational leaflets. Then, they went around local villages, donating basic hand hygiene kits to village groups and delivering health promotion messages. They would send me photos of these moving ceremonies where they would hand over the gifts to grateful recipients.

I found it overwhelming. How could our differences be so big? Ultimately, Malawi was probably well suited to managing Covid in some ways: an outdoors society, a young population, and homes that were extremely well-ventilated. Nevertheless, they did experience significant loss and major economic disruption, with all the health impacts that would naturally follow.

During my last visit to Sydney, we talked about his dreams for the future. Education was always central; he thought there was no path for development in Malawi that didn't start with education, and he wanted to create a teachers' training college and then, ultimately, another university. But he also now wanted to create a primary care clinic in his area, hoping that emerging health challenges could be better identified and treated before they escalated and became life-defining.

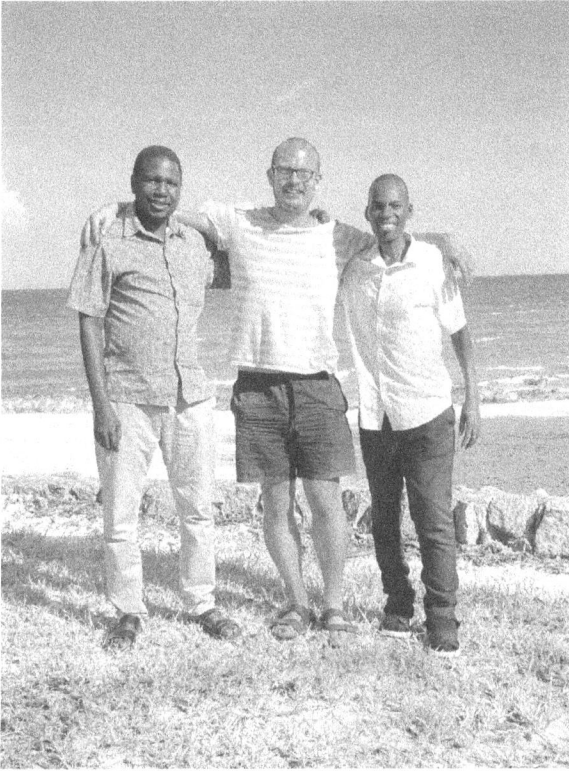

With a fading Sydney (right) and Feston Singoyi on the shores of Lake Malawi.

I arrived to see Sydney on the 24th of November 2021. One day after my arrival, South Africa announced the discovery of what was quickly named Omicron, a new, seemingly highly transmissible variant of Covid. This time, the UK and much of the world reacted rapidly. South Africa and a number of countries in Southern Africa were placed on the UK's red list; a day later, Malawi was added.

I had to leave Malawi as quickly as possible.

Nervous that I risked being stuck in the country where only tiny numbers of international flights were coming in (even before these announcements) and managing some stressful

Kafkaesque bureaucracy – both British and Malawian – I managed to book a quarantine hotel, get a Covid test, and fly home.

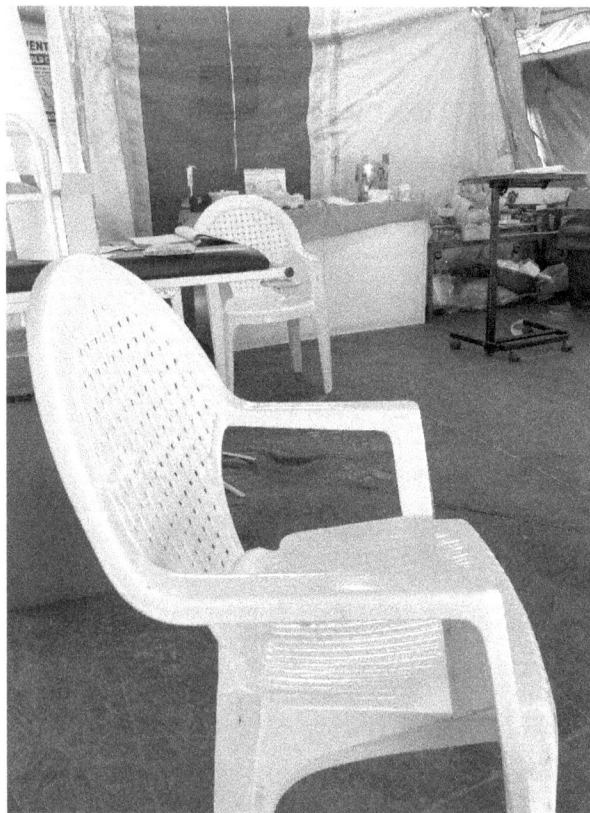

My Covid test centre.

Even finding a Covid test proved eye-opening. In the UK, it couldn't have been easier to get one; every neighbourhood had somewhere you could go. In Malawi, however, few people travel or had any other particular reason to know their Covid status, and there were few places in the country to test. Fortunately, one was about an hour from where I was staying, a small dilapidated tent on the site of Mzuzu Hospital in Northern Malawi. It comprised a bed and a couple of plastic chairs. I got my test, and the results arrived just in time for me to be allowed onto my departure flight at Lilongwe airport and the journey home.

Back at Heathrow, I was met by security and had my passport confiscated. It prompted a viscerally uncomfortable feeling, which gave me a fleeting insight into the lack of agency and powerlessness that many in our society feel on a long-term or permanent basis when dealing with authorities. At my Covid hotel – my new home for 11 days – a perfectly comfortable room overlooked one of Heathrow's runways.

Fortunately, work would keep me busy. No sooner had the borders been largely closed to Southern African countries, with all the economic impacts to them, than it became clear that Omicron was spreading quickly and was all over the UK.

Over the next 11 days, I found myself doing eerily familiar work from my unusual surroundings of a hotel room: attending briefings with the chief medical officer and UKHSA (the successor to Public Health England) to try to understand the emerging science of the new variants and its impact; briefing colleagues, local politicians and community members about what was going on; working with my team to get advice out among the community; and trying to work out whether there was anything else I thought we should be doing in this new context.

Omicron was spreading super-fast. The early thinking was that it might not be as severe as previous variants, and with the population widely vaccinated at this point, there was a logic that its impact would be limited. My instincts were to reinforce basic safety precautions and to keep focusing on reaching people who weren't fully vaccinated, but otherwise to allow people to get on with their lives. Society had been disrupted enough, and unless the evidence emerged that

Omicron was actually more dangerous than initially thought, we needed to ride this one out.

I was allowed out of my room to walk around the hotel car park for 20-25 minutes per day. On my first afternoon of "yard time", I had an idea. With ten more days in quarantine, if I ran 4.2 km around the car park each day, I would complete a marathon. With images of Captain Tom, the centenarian whose garden walk raised over £30 million, and other slightly madcap (and less famous and lucrative) Covid isolation fundraisers in my head, maybe I could put my enforced quarantine to good use and raise some money to take forward one of Sydney's dreams. Sydney and Feston had shown me a plot of land they hoped to purchase to build a teacher training college and, one day, a university. I set a ridiculously ambitious target of £20,000… enough to buy the land.

Each day, I did my run (around 70 laps of the car park) and reported my efforts on social media. I ended up being interviewed on BBC Five Live and Channel 5 TV, and sponsored by seemingly everyone I had ever known: from friends to people in Newham, colleagues in public health and my professional past, and dozens of complete strangers. Amazingly, on my last day in quarantine, I hit my target!

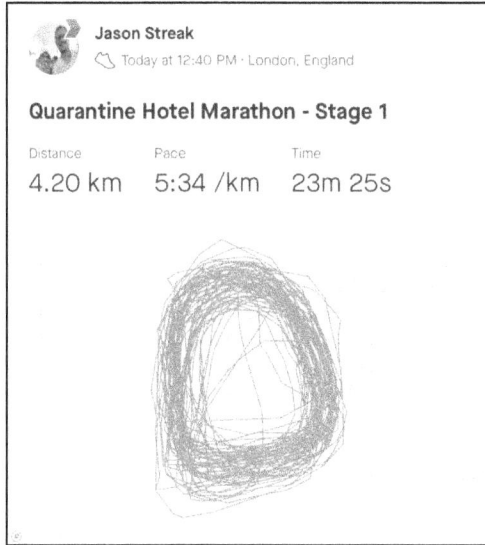

Quarantine Hotel Marathon Strava.

It was a particularly strange two weeks in what had been a very strange two years. The emotions of saying goodbye to a dear friend, the confrontation with basic Malawian healthcare, being caught up in forced public health measures myself, the oddness of managing a pandemic from a hotel room, and the joy of my successful quarantine marathon.

Lying with my thoughts, there was so much to reflect upon in the hotel bed at night. In particular, I thought constantly about the two very different worlds I had been in. My day job is tackling the deep inequalities in health within Newham, and between our population in the East End of London and much of the country. But global inequalities run far deeper. While we lend ventilators from our TV programmes to our hospitals, in Malawi we hand out buckets and soap to committed community members as the first line of defence. We talk about the aforementioned "Inverse Care Law" to describe how those who need the best healthcare are least likely to have it. That truth operates within the UK, even with our universal National Health Service, but operates so much more powerfully when we think globally.

The pandemic highlighted that this is not just a moral issue, though it is clearly so. While those in wealthy countries get themselves as fully vaccinated as possible, do we leave enough in the system – both in terms of vaccines and the resources to deliver them – for the countries that can't buy their way to the front of the queue? With the risk of new variants, vaccine resistance, or particular severity, if people are unvaccinated anywhere, we are at risk everywhere.

My connection to our work in Malawi remains as strong as ever. In 2024, in Northern Malawi, the primary care clinic was opened in Sydney's memory, providing basic healthcare to the local community, and the first brick was laid for Kunyanja Teacher Training College.

Chapter 17
Permacrisis

When the Omicron variant appeared, things could be seen as glass half-full or half-empty. Pessimistically, the rapid spread of this new variant, which had travelled internationally at high speed (leaving my hotel quarantine experience essentially redundant) and its reach into a population already relatively exposed to previous variants, was just another reminder of the risks that emerging viruses pose in a globalised world.

Omicron emerged from a relatively unvaccinated part of the world and gave clear evidence of the need to ensure global protection against vaccine-preventable infectious diseases. The speed at which this variant spread gave credence to the criticism that dates back to John Snow's foundational removal of the tap from the water pump in Soho, namely, public health action sometimes shuts the stable door long after the horse has bolted. In this case, we were literally guarding the stable door, and the microscopic horses snuck out right in front of our eyes.

As many have cautioned in the period since, including Sir Patrick Vallance, the UK government's chief scientific advisor throughout the Covid period, future pandemics in our globalised, unequal world are inevitable. It is a matter of when, not if. That central idea of risk (as well as the many benefits) of our interconnected, mutually dependent, globalised world would soon be brought out in other powerful ways.

The glass half-full interpretation, however, was that as much as we had undeniably witnessed the rapid spread of Omicron, we came through it comparatively unscathed. The clinical impacts of the Omicron variant were much more limited than previous waves. In our largely immunised population in the UK, the vaccine held, and fatality and wider hospitalisation rates were far below previous levels.

The link between infection and serious illness had been significantly weakened. Moreover, it was clear at this point that the rapidly developed vaccine technologies were highly adaptable to new strains, and the mechanisms of vaccine production and distribution meant that, if necessary, vaccine scientists and pharmaceutical companies could respond quickly to genetic variations.

I came out of that period feeling more upbeat. While we were always aware of the possibilities of vaccine-resistant strains and new emergent viral threats, it definitely felt that – building on the success of the vaccine programme over the preceding 12 months – we had reached the next stage of the end of the pandemic.

It was still another year before the WHO – on May 5th 2023 – announced that the global health emergency, declared three and a half years earlier, was now over. By then, the world's attention had already long moved on; that week, in the UK at least, it was local elections and the coronation of King Charles which held the attention of the evening news.

Our focus had shifted professionally and more widely in society long before May 5th. I remember chatting with colleagues about the pub nights we looked forward to when everything was over; the opportunities to let down our increasingly greying hair and celebrate our work during the pandemic. We did make it to the pub occasionally, but never specifically to acknowledge the journey and *the end*. Just as we were emerging from Omicron and recognising that we were moving to a better place vis-à-vis Covid, other enormous challenges started rapidly appearing.

On February 24th 2022, only a couple of months after the Omicron scare, Russia invaded Ukraine. This was the most significant attack by one independent country against another in Europe since the Second World War. It was scary. Much as the first wave of Covid hit Italy, a country similar to our own in many ways, we were now witnessing a belligerent power sending missiles, tanks, and soldiers towards cities like Kyiv and Kharkiv. Cities full of vibrant modern European urban life – beautiful architecture, bars and restaurants, thriving culture and universities – were turned into war zones.

Quite apart from the general concern for people caught up in what seemed like a totally unnecessary conflict, the impact began to ripple into our home lives very quickly.

Domestic energy prices had already increased as the world emerged out of lockdown and economic demand rose. However, the Russian invasion caused a further sharp shock due to disruptions in supply, alongside sanctions and embargo regimes. Suddenly, global events 2,000 miles away profoundly impacted people's ability to make ends meet at home. Talk of a cost of living crisis began as people, who had just about managed previously, were now facing the prospect of being unable to heat their homes. Rents were also rising, and inflation – which had remained low for a long time, mitigating the impact of the stagnating wages most people were experiencing – started to rise.

Six months later, there was another unexpected external shock. A new scandal had taken hold in the political news. It emerged that, for months throughout the pandemic, there were regular parties attended by politicians, advisors, and government officials in 10 Downing Street, the Prime Minister's home and office. It is hard to imagine what this breach of trust would have meant if news had come out in the middle of the pandemic; the Dominic Cummings incident was trivial by comparison. Coming towards the end of the pandemic, it caused a major breakdown in public trust and support for the government and the pandemic Prime Minister, Boris Johnson, was forced to resign.

Liz Truss became Prime Minister on the 5th of September 2022 and appointed Kwasi Kwarteng as Chancellor of the Exchequer.

Two weeks later, the new government made a major set of economic announcements in a mini-budget, lighting another rocket under the cost of living crisis. Inflation was now rapidly increasing, interest rates were climbing, and with them came much higher costs in housing, both for those with mortgages and even more for renters. Food prices were surging, too.

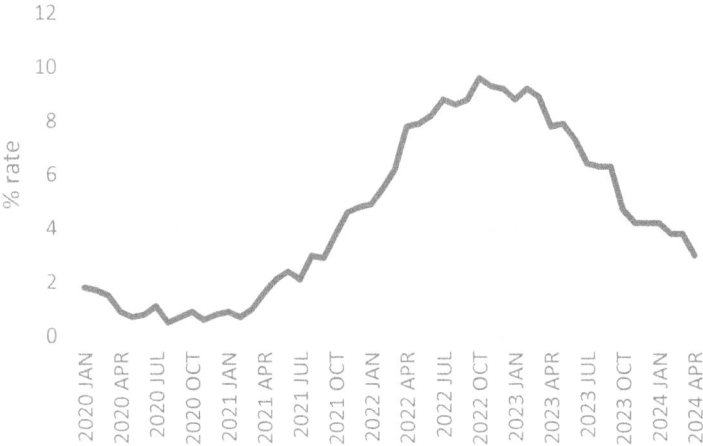

Trend in inflation (Consumer Price Index), January 2020-April 2024. Source: Office for National Statistics.

Few, if anyone, will not have noticed the rising prices from 2022-2024. However, the challenge of balancing household budgets became incredibly hard for those managing on low to moderate incomes. For many, the proportion of household income spent on the absolute basics – housing (rent or mortgage), energy and food – reached simply unsustainable levels. In many working households, poverty grew, as did the use of food banks. Homelessness became a growing outcome for families who could previously cope. With wages still low and many people on the lowest wages struggling to find more work hours, or juggling work and caring responsibilities, the cost of living crisis exerted a vice-like grip.

In Newham, where there was significant underlying socioeconomic vulnerability pre-pandemic, the impact of this was profound. Whilst the pandemic had created a surge in collective responses – from national policy decisions to extraordinary local collective action – the response on both levels to rising costs was much less ambitious and far-reaching.

At a national level, the combined fiscal impact of the pandemic and the Truss/Kwarteng budget, allied to a more fragmented sense of national purpose, meant the safety net – which had been strengthened profoundly during the height of the pandemic – was being taken apart.

Most widely recognised as part of the Covid safety net was the Coronavirus job retention programme known as the furlough scheme: an unparalleled policy intervention that safeguarded people's jobs and livelihoods while the economy ground to a halt. The furlough scheme, combined with support for self-employed people through this period, saw an investment of close to £100 billion to support people's living standards. Indeed, it was of huge importance in Newham where, at one stage in the heart of the pandemic, close to 100,000 people (out of a working-age population of around 250,000) were supported by the furlough scheme or social security benefits.

There were also other hugely important policy interventions during the pandemic to support those struggling the most, including our most vulnerable residents.

Early on, a policy called "Everyone In" gave local areas the support needed to help get homeless people off the street. Before Covid, in Newham, we had a significant challenge of rough sleeping, particularly around a certain shopping centre in Stratford, close to the Olympic Park, which had become an unofficial and incredibly dangerous informal homeless shelter. Before Covid, we had seen flyers shared overseas which had identified this exceedingly busy shopping centre – filled with the usual high street shops from Sainsbury's to Boots and Sports Direct, as well as a longstanding market – as a good "first destination" for people arriving in London. We had already made some headway in prioritising more therapeutic support to help people get off the streets, but "Everyone In" gave us the impetus and money from central government needed to move much faster.

During the pandemic, we were able to support those with "no recourse to public funds", including visa overstayers who were remaining in the UK. In around two weeks in March 2020, we were able to help nearly 200 homeless people move into accommodation and support them to a life off the streets. Since then, we have supported thousands of people – just in Newham, alone – and never returned to the previous high levels. The situation is becoming ever more challenging, however, as I will touch on below.

Alongside "Everyone In", a profoundly impactful policy of the Covid period was the "eviction ban", also introduced in March 2020. It gave tenants of both social and privately rented housing various rights through an extended period of the pandemic, protecting them from eviction by their landlords. The eviction ban stopped an inevitable uptick in homelessness, causing heartache for the families impacted and major challenges for local government trying to support rehousing while trying to manage the infection's spread.

The lifting of the eviction ban in June 2021 – coming at the time it did – opened the floodgates to homelessness. This was not just affecting people with multiple vulnerabilities (such as those with drug or alcohol dependency, very poor mental health, or a lack of immigration rights); for many, this new housing affordability crisis was about poverty and an inability to manage to live on modest incomes. The workforce in Newham includes many people doing the work that keeps our cities going; their incomes were not keeping pace with rapidly rising rents and other prices, though.

Another policy that had been implemented during the pandemic had an unexpected origin. In the 2000s, when I had worked on child poverty policy, we had often discussed the challenge of "cutting through" with campaign messages to the general public. Much of the British public thinks of poverty as a feature of Britain from past times – a Victorian or Dickensian representation – or something that only exists in developing countries. The concept of relative poverty (i.e., needing enough money to participate even at a basic level) in an affluent society just doesn't resonate with many people. Professional campaigners or politicians often appear to struggle to find a message that resonates with the wider public.

We would often discuss the need for authentic voices to communicate the issue in a manner that more effectively connected with the public. But we found those voices hard to come by. Poverty is both stigmatising and disempowering. As a society, we blame the poor for their situation, quick to judge people for not taking advantage of what society has to offer and for not "pulling themselves up by their bootstraps". Few seemed willing to step into that fray.

But during the pandemic, the Manchester United and England striker Marcus Rashford started to. In only a short number of years, he had gone from being a child whose mum worked multiple jobs and missed meals to make ends meet, to a multi-millionaire footballer. He was by far the most impactful advocate on child poverty I had ever heard in a UK context.

Among many interventions, in September 2021, he said:

"The entire nation got behind the national team this summer, so let's put these figures in football terms: You can fill 27 Wembley stadiums with the 2.5 million children that are struggling to know where their next meal might be coming from today.

What is it going to take for these children to be prioritised?

Instead of removing support through social security, we should be focusing efforts on developing a sustainable long-term road map out of this child hunger pandemic."[29]

What was amazing was not simply that he put his head above the parapet (very unusual for sporting celebrities in the UK) but that he sought to influence policy and call for system change. His advocacy had a huge impact, with local authorities receiving resources like Holiday Activity Funds and Household Support Funds, offering additional basic safety nets in local areas.

But now, as we moved from the pandemic to a multi-pronged cost of living crisis, ambitious policies to support people against poverty and homelessness through the pandemic years were fraying. As a local authority during the pandemic, we had been forced to prioritise actions and stop doing certain things. In doing so, we created an extra corps of staff who contributed to the collective effort. (In the community, this was also true where the furlough scheme had allowed many people to get involved with volunteering.) But now, obviously, life was getting back to normal; people had their own jobs, their normal lives to focus on, and council staff returned to their primary roles.

---

[29] Marcus Rashford says child food poverty 'devastatingly' worse. BBC News, 6 September 2021.

The change was about more than capacity, however. The pandemic had been a moment of collective focus and effort, but as we moved beyond the pandemic's most challenging times, our goals fragmented to a more normal pre-Covid place, where responsibilities and concerns became more diffuse. There was no longer a single burning issue to get behind.

Meanwhile, the longstanding challenge of financial austerity in local government returned after a brief pause; we were back in a world of rising demand and diminished resources, and now had to deal with a spectrum of challenges compounded by the cost of living crisis. People in the community and community groups had to focus on a wider set of priorities.

Alongside the cost of living crisis came a seemingly endless series of challenges; some related to that, others as legacies of the pandemic or independent of it.

- The Ukraine invasion, for example, led to the Homes for Ukraine scheme, where the UK government incentivised people to host those fleeing the conflict. This had a symbiotic relationship with the initial spike in public consciousness and concern. At the same time, there were large increases in refugees and asylum seekers from many other parts of the world. Suddenly, multiple hotels in our borough were being block-booked by subcontractors of the Home Office.

- As mentioned already, the cost of living crisis and the end of pandemic support led to a homelessness crisis. In Newham, where large numbers of people were just about managing on low to moderate incomes but living in the private rented sector, rapidly increasing rents were becoming unaffordable. People in huge numbers were presenting as homeless to the local authority.

- The NHS and social care were facing enormous challenges. The combination of Covid itself, the cancellation of considerable numbers of health procedures, and general difficulty in accessing basic healthcare during the pandemic led to a crisis in healthcare. We had many unwell people, a service with too much demand, and a burned-out workforce.
- New infection scares appeared; the spread of the MPox virus (previously known as monkeypox), concerns about polio (long since disappeared from the UK, but traces starting to appear in countries that hadn't seen polio for years), and a surge in measles as vaccination levels in some parts of the community had reach dangerously low levels.

These challenges hit a public sector running on fumes, and now failing many people. Years of underinvestment, compounded by the challenges of Covid to people's wellbeing, resulted in a surge of poor health.

Global interconnectedness and global instability have given this period a feeling of permanent crisis. We have chronic challenges of longstanding inequality, a reduced safety net, and severely weakened social infrastructure. These chronic conditions are highly problematic for our population's wellbeing on their own, but also leave us incredibly vulnerable to acute crises, ranging from war to new infection threats.

If resilience is the ability to bend but not break, these combined conditions have shown that our collective resilience only goes so far. Covid was a profound challenge, and while it left lasting damage for so many, it didn't crush us because of the way we supported each other, from state investment in the safety net to community collective action to interpersonal support. It is perhaps inevitable that the response to an acute crisis is different to the chronic challenges that we face daily, yet the imbalance seems disproportionate. Our lack of investment in the social infrastructure that builds that resilience leaves society weaker overall and less prepared for when the next disaster hits.

Chapter 18
Conclusion

Covid turned our world upside down. It was a remarkable time, a period when society operated in fundamentally different ways from what we had taken for granted previously. Faced with such a significant acute health risk, the resilience of society was put to the test. While many were severely impacted – from loss of life and loved ones, to the long-term health effects of Long Covid, to the economic and social scars of the steps taken to manage the pandemic – society also responded amazingly, from the brilliance of the vaccine creators to the persistence and generosity of community volunteers.

Now, with Covid very much in the background, we have returned to the place where pandemics sit as just one item on the global risk register, a risk register feeling ever lengthy and daunting.

Of course, it is possible that a new variant can emerge at any time, a variant that is both highly transmissible and highly harmful despite the levels of population vaccination. If that happens, we will return to some of the most challenging days of the pandemic.

But, for now, we can look back and reflect.

What are the lessons we need to take from this chapter in our lives, soon to pass into public health history? At some point, the UK government's pandemic public inquiry will eventually be reported fully. It will have plenty to say about pandemic readiness, from surveillance to PPE, global cooperation, vaccination, and more. I will leave those conclusions to the inquiry and the inevitable debate surrounding its conclusion.

My focus, by contrast, is what we learned from our pandemic experience for non-pandemic times, from the everyday challenges of chronic inequalities to the relationship between state and community, to the connection between central and local government, and the nature of resilient places.

The Powerful Combination of Civil Society and an Enabling State

The pandemic showed how the state – both centrally and locally – when willing to trust and believe in the power of community, can achieve far more than acting independently. Whether in the work we did to try to ensure no one went hungry or lonely, to make testing widely available, or to reach many who may otherwise not have been vaccinated, an active partnership between a committed local state and bottom-up community activity made a huge difference.

Local government – thinking about the population as a whole – could play a huge role as a facilitator for any number of public health initiatives, with its democratic mandate, the power of convening and coordinating, and the ability to build capacity in the community even when funding is limited. This is true both in quantitative and qualitative terms.

Undoubtedly, the sheer scale of people reached during Covid far exceeded what we would have reached through a purely state-based system. Building capacity unlocked thousands of hours of volunteer time through community groups and faith organisations, but it also ensured that we reached *more people* as we overcame the tenuous or non-existent connections many people have with statutory services.

This approach was also about listening. Our connections gave us an ear to the ground, hearing daily about the challenges residents were experiencing, enabling us to adapt and augment our responses as we went forward. This isn't about the hollowing out of the state (nor abrogating responsibility to the community) but about the collaborative and enabling state working together with communities with common purpose.

The state will never have the resources or capabilities to meet population needs, nor will it create the trust and connections to get close to all parts of the community. As I have touched upon at length, the pandemic, in common with other disasters, created a sense of a common goal and spirit that brought people together. Should that not be our purpose all of the time?

Not Losing the Microscope on Inequalities

We have long known of the broad links between inequalities and health outcomes, but during the pandemic, we saw in real-time the myriad ways that inequalities shape people's lives and lead to worse health outcomes. There were inequalities in who could work from home, travel by car, isolate at home, shop online, access health information, isolate from work when required, and navigate remote learning. Without trying to address these issues, our communities remained exposed to ever more disproportionate risk. Infection control in communities like Newham, therefore, meant trying to address subjects like food security, labour rights, immigration advice, household overcrowding, and digital access. If we are serious about tackling the social determinants of health, these kinds of issues need to remain central to our approach.

The pandemic also revealed that racial and ethnic inequalities in health (which had been peripheral in the discussion of health inequalities for too long) played second fiddle to analysis based on a socio-economic lens. The coincidence of the Black Lives Matter protests and evidence on the disproportionate impact the pandemic had on Black and Asian populations forced a significant pause and reflection, and gave fresh momentum for addressing these issues. Our work, particularly on vaccination, showed that both the challenges and the opportunities to address inequalities start with *listening* to the concerns of impacted communities. While the social determinants of health matter deeply, the pandemic also showed that with the right approaches, based on deep intentionality and purpose, and the thoughtful application of evidence and resources to local context, we can make a profound difference. There is a long journey ahead.

The Importance of Locally-Informed and Locally Delivered Policy

Another area where the pandemic shone a bright light – but which has been a feature of policymaking discussion for years – is how policy is determined centrally in Britain. Far too often, policy is developed in Whitehall without enough understanding of the granularity and complexity on the ground or the different needs of different places. In real-time, we saw the disconnect, with centrally-made decisions having limited or differential impact at a local level and varying with local context.

The challenge for policymakers is twofold. Where policy is being made centrally, it is vital to ensure that it is being made by those who really understand the realities on the ground, the challenges of delivery, what is likely to work and what is not, what barriers exist to a policy working effectively, and how to deliver in such a way that makes a difference. It requires feedback loops so that policy adapts and evolves to the reality of delivery. Although centralised British policymaking is a barrier, it shouldn't be hard to fix. It was easy to see that when policymakers engaged more deeply with us locally, their decisions were more informed and, therefore, more effective. It's hardly rocket science.

The next stage is a bit harder, but equally a challenge worth rising to. How can we devolve policymaking further, to a local level, so that areas can be effectively resourced for their different needs? How can decision-making be more responsive to the different needs of different communities?

Foundations of Resilient Places

Whether to support people through the challenges posed by chronic risks or to enable effective responses when disaster strikes, the underlying *resilience* that exists in a place is a major determinant of our ability to support each other, particularly the most vulnerable.

Many factors of place contribute to that resilience, and some key factors relate to policy choice:

- The state of public services, like health and education.

- Strong local democratic institutions, able to respond with agility and humanity.

- Community resources – from places of worship to libraries – which can act as anchors for people, where support can be mobilised, and safety can be sought.

- Partnerships of trust where local leaders, from politicians to community champions, can come together around common goals.

However, these have been severely weakened through years of austerity and multiple crises. Rebuilding the combined social infrastructure of a place is vital if we're going to be able to respond to the many challenges that lie ahead. According to the Institute for Fiscal Studies,[30] local government in the UK in the most deprived areas has 35% less funding per person than 15 years ago. With less funding in areas like

---

[30] How have English councils' funding and spending changed? 2010 to 2024, Kate Ogden and David Phillips, *Institute for Fiscal Studies*, June 2024

health and education, how can we respond to the social challenges we face?

It can be tempting to judge our success in responding to the challenges of Covid, or ongoing issues such as poverty and inequality, by the array of initiatives we implemented and the particular outcomes those initiatives achieved. There are so many things to be proud of about our pandemic response, both across the country and in Newham. But it is equally important to look at the big picture... how effective were we in totality, how many lives were positively impacted by our cumulative actions, and how many lives were severely impacted by Covid despite our actions? These impacts include loss of life, livelihood, education, physical health, and mental health.

The pandemic may be over, but its legacy remains strong for many, compounded by the crises that have followed closely on its heels. Inequalities, so often assumed to be simply part of our reality, are those different boats that give people differential shelter through these storms. Some benefit from an ocean liner, insulated almost entirely from whatever the world throws at them. There are sturdy ships that may rock from side to side, and occasionally have accidents, but which provide shelter for much of our country. For too many others, however, fragile sea crafts are all that is on offer; they provide all but the flimsiest protection from the crashing waves and winds. Our pandemic response from national policy to local action showed an ability to at least buttress these crafts, providing some cover, but it ultimately comes down to political will and collective purpose if we want to house the whole population in the strongest vessels. If there is one lesson, more than any other, I have taken away from the pandemic, it's that if these explicit commitments exist, we can do extraordinary things. Let's not wait for another crisis before we rise to that challenge.

Other Books from the Publisher

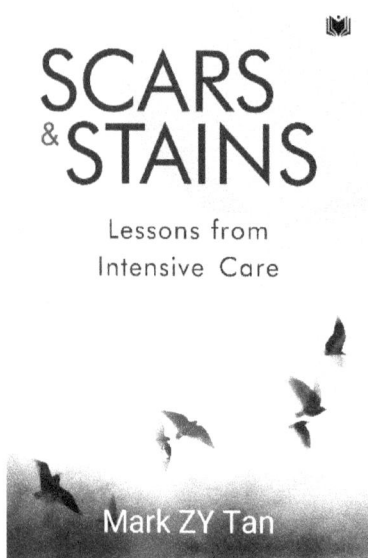

Scars & Stains: Lessons from Intensive Care

Airway. Breathing. Circulation. Disability. Exposure.

Perhaps the five most misunderstood words in life support.

Join anaesthetics and intensive care doctor, and award-winning writer Dr Mark ZY Tan, as he lays bare the clinical, ethical, and moral dilemmas facing intensive care professionals in today's complex world. *Scars and Stains* takes readers into the world of intensive care – including the Covid pandemic – where split-second decisions and precise skills can forever impact the lives of patients and their families. It is a journey that crosses continents, communities, and cultures – from the slums of Thailand and jungles of Papua New Guinea to the wealthiest districts of London and largest hospitals in the UK. Caring for some of the most unwell patients, with the help of high-tech machinery, and often in emotionally volatile situations, Mark provides moving – and often eye-opening – insights into this fascinating frontier of medicine. He brings together the science underpinning this high-stakes specialty with the humanity required to navigate life and death decisions.

Written for anyone interested in the reality of life on the frontline, the book challenges preconceived notions of the ICU, sheds light on the often-misunderstood realities faced by patients, their loved ones, and healthcare professionals in the most challenging of environments, and guides readers in considering their own preferences and priorities when faced with life-limiting illnesses.

Foreword by Matt Morgan, author of Critical (2020) and One Medicine (2023)

Patients First: How to Save The NHS

This life-saving prescription should be widely debated by all who care about our nation's most vital institution.
Simon Stevens, former Chief Executive of NHS England

PATIENTS FIRST

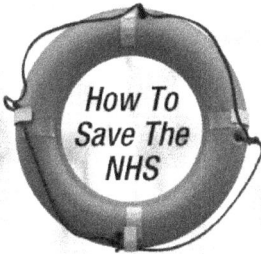

How To Save The NHS

Leslie Turnberg

In *Patients First*, Leslie Turnberg, former President of the Royal College of Physicians, focuses on the needs of NHS patients and the staff who care for them. Shining a light on the many challenges facing the NHS and Primary and Social Care, and resisting any suggestion of yet another wholesale reorganisation, he pinpoints where and how to improve outcomes.

It is clear that the caring services must change and a patient-centred model – where a disillusioned workforce is brought back into satisfying and contented employment – should be the aim. Chapters on Social care and Primary Care come first, as so much in secondary care is dependent on them. Chapters on Public Health, Mental Health, and Maternity

Care provide examples of where significant improvements may be gained. Further chapters on Trust in the NHS, Research, and Funding follow.

Patients First is a must-read for anyone interested in an NHS action plan for the future.

Lord Turnberg carefully takes the temperature of an ailing NHS. His life-saving prescription should be widely debated by all who care about our nation's most vital institution. **Lord Simon Stevens, former Chief Executive of NHS England**

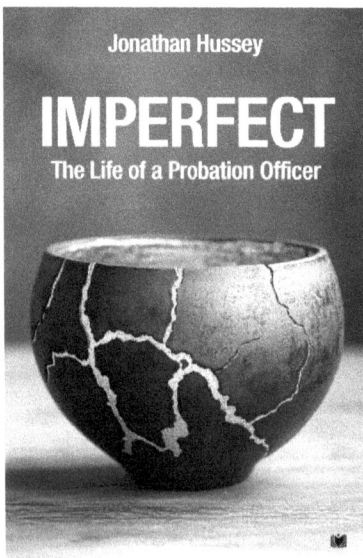

Imperfect: The Life of a Probation Officer

In *Imperfect*, Jonathan Hussey — author of *Reoffending* and the *Probation Workbook* series — offers a compelling and unflinching memoir of his two decades working within the Criminal Justice System.

Spanning his early years in adult probation to his time in youth justice and through the turbulent rollout of Transforming Rehabilitation, Jonathan reflects on the wide range of individuals he has worked with — from repeat offenders and sex offenders to young people on the cusp of change. With honesty and insight, he explores not just the professional challenges but the emotional toll the job can take if not managed correctly, pulling back the curtain on the mental health pressures that working in probation can bring about.

Imperfect is more than a personal story — it's a reflective, eye-opening guide for those considering a career in probation, current practitioners navigating a complex system, or anyone drawn to the realities behind one of society's most demanding and misunderstood public service roles. Blending personal narrative with professional reflection, Jonathan captures both the frustrations and the redemptive power of working with complex individuals.

Thought-provoking, honest, and deeply human, *Imperfect* is essential reading for anyone interested in probation careers, offender rehabilitation, criminal justice in general, or the personal impact of frontline public service work.

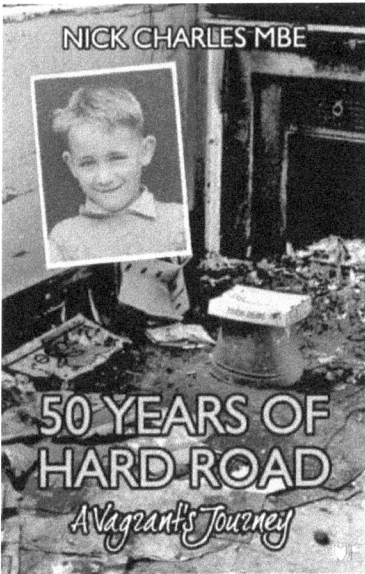

50 Years of Hard Road: A Vagrant's Journey

Nick Charles MBE is a pioneer in treating alcohol dependency. As the founder of both the Chaucer Clinic and the Gainsborough Foundation, he was the first person to be honoured by the Queen 'for services to people with alcohol problems' and his work – over four decades – has helped tens of thousands of people. But Nick's decorated success overlays an extraordinary and unforgettable personal journey, for Nick was once an alcoholic vagrant sleeping rough on the streets of London.

In *50 Years of Hard Road*, Nick details his time in the abyss of alcohol addiction; a period that despatched relationships, his health, his career, and so much more. Forced to live on the streets for four years, Nick recalls the tough times, the characters he met, and the ever-present call of alcohol, but also how he slowly built up two carrier bags-worth of painstaking research into alcohol and its effects on his fellow man. It was through the documents in these carrier bags that Nick's life was to change forever when, in the mid-1970s, he was taken under the wing of a doctor who cared for those on skid row. This dedicated medic recognised the treasure trove of information Nick had developed.

50 Years of Hard Road is a remarkable, uplifting, and often humorous story of one man's journey from the depths of life-crushing alcohol dependency, to running alcohol clinics and programmes across the country. It describes an incredible life filled with high points, low points, and amazing adventures in-between.